T0210685

When Things Go Wrong In Urology

Faiz Motiwala · Hanif Motiwala
Sanchia S. Goonewardene
Editors

When Things Go Wrong In Urology

Reflections to Improve Practice

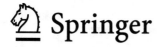
Springer

Editors
Faiz Motiwala
Queen Elizabeth Hospital
London, UK

Hanif Motiwala
Southend University Hospital
Westcliff-on-Sea, UK

Sanchia S. Goonewardene
Princess Alexandra Hospital
Harlow, Essex, UK

ISBN 978-3-031-13660-3   ISBN 978-3-031-13658-0   (eBook)
https://doi.org/10.1007/978-3-031-13658-0

This Springer imprint is published by the registered company Springer Nature Switzerland AG
The registered company address is: Gewerbestrasse 11, 6330 Cham, Switzerland

Preface

Welcome to *When things go Wrong in Urology*.

On behalf of my team and I, it has been a pleasure putting this together for you. This is an important topic for both patients and clinicians alike and is specifically written for you. We are lucky to have experts from around the world contributing to this book. A myriad of problems can create issues for healthcare professionals. This book looks at and brings together issues that are of a difficult nature. These include clinical negligence and malpractice, medicolegal pitfalls, communication, digital communication, legal records, consent, administrative problems, diagnostics, operating theatre issues, human factors in health care, managing difficult seniors, leadership in medicine, managing a complaint, how to avoid failure, raising a concern in training, managing a GMC investigation, approach to a GMC investigation, and burn out in medicine.

The key is to put the care of your patient first—do this and you will always succeed.

With Best Wishes.

Birmingham, UK   Faiz Motiwala
Southend-on-Sea, UK   Hanif Motiwala
Harlow, UK   Sanchia S. Goonewardene

Acknowledgements

For my family and friends—always supporting me in what I do.
For all the superheroes in my life—you are truly inspirational.
For my team at Springer Nature, for always giving me a chance to get published.
For all the amazing clinicians who contributed to this book.

Contents

About the Editors

Faiz Motiwala Faiz Motiwala qualified from the Peninsula College of Medicine and Dentistry. He completed his master's degree in Surgical Sciences from the University of Edinburgh alongside his Foundation Years and Core Surgical Training. He has contributed chapters to the 'Core Surgical Procedures for Urology Trainees'. He has presented at several conferences around the world including Dubai, and after qualifying he visited Sudan to do voluntary work.

Hanif Motiwala Mr. Motiwala is well known to the community worldwide. He was Professor of Urology in India and has also served as an FRCS Urol Examiner. He has been the Training Programme Director for the London Deanery, Imperial Rotation, and was well liked by all of his trainees. He has also been a Lecturer at the Institute of Urology and Oxford Trainees.

He has over 25 years' experience as a Consultant in Urology and extensive exposure to senior leadership roles in healthcare provision and professional institutions including Chairman of the surgical division at Wexham Park Hospital. He also has a strong track record of achieving clinical targets within tightly controlled budgets, developing innovative strategies to improve patient care and optimise the use of resources, for which he received a Bronze Award.

He is a dedicated and committed surgeon, utilising teaching, surgical, and medical skills for the greater good through international voluntary work, building capability and skills in reconstructive surgery in India and Africa. He was conferred a position as Visiting Professor—University of Khartoum, Sudan, 2009 in recognition of voluntary work in Sudan, conducting final Urology Examinations to train qualified surgeons, providing training to surgeons in reconstruction, and carrying out complex surgery.

Sanchia S. Goonewardene Sanchia Goonewardene qualified from Birmingham Medical School with Honours in Clinical Science and a BMedSc Degree in Medical Genetics and Molecular Medicine. She has a specific interest in academia during her spare time, with over 764 publications to her name with 2 papers as a number 1 most cited in fields (Biomedical Library) and has significantly contributed to the Urological Academic World—she has since added a section to the European Association of Urology Congress on Prostate Cancer Survivorship and Supportive

Care and has been an associate member of an EAU guidelines panel on Chronic Pelvic Pain. She has also been asked to Abstract Review for EAU and EMUC and is a member of the YAU-ERUS board. She has been the UK lead in an EAU led study on Salvage Prostatectomy. She has also contributed to the BURST IDENTIFY study as a collaborator.

Her background with research entails an MPhil, the work from which went on to be drawn up as a document for PCUK then, NICE endorsed. She gained funding from the Wellcome Trust for her Research Elective. She is also an Alumni of the Urology Foundation, who sponsored a trip to USANZ trainee week. She also has 9 books published—*Core Surgical Procedures for Urology Trainees (Ranked 3rd in Book Authorities' 100 Greatest Urology Books of All Time), Prostate Cancer Survivorship, Basic Urological Management, Management of Non-Muscle Invasive Bladder Cancer, Salvage Therapy in Prostate Cancer, Muscle Invasive Bladder Cancer, Surgical Strategies for Endourology for Stones, Mens' Health and Wellbeing*, and *Robotic Surgery for Renal Cancer.*

She has supervised her first thesis with King's College London and Guys Hospital, (BMedSci Degree -first class, students' thesis score-95%). She has Associate Editor position with the Journal of Robotic Surgery and is responsible as Urology Section Editor. She is an Editorial board member of the World Journal of Urology. She was invited to be Guest Editor for a Special Issue on Salvage Therapy in Prostate Cancer. She is also a review board member for BMJ case reports. She has taught for both Royal College of Surgeons, RCS Edinburgh and England, is currently an MSc Tutor at the University of Edinburgh and Royal College of Surgeons of Edinburgh Surgical Sciences course, has also been an MSc Thesis marker for them, and prepared written exam questions for the MSc course.

Additionally, she is on The International Continence Society Panel on Pelvic Floor Dysfunction which has developed an international document and core document for ICS; she also contributed to a webinar on Pelvic Floor Dysfunction on Pelvic Floor Dysfunction, Good Urodynamic Practice Panel; she is an ICS abstract reviewer and has been an EPoster Chair at ICS.

More recently, she has been an ICS Ambassador and is an ICS Mentor. She has also chaired semi-live surgery at YAU-ERUS and presented her work as part of the Young Academic Urology Section at ERUS.

Abbreviations

A&E	Accident and Emergency
AES	Approved Education Supervisor
AKI	Acute Kidney Injury
ARCP	Annual Review of Curriculum Progress
BAME	Black and Minority Ethnic
BAUS	British Association of Urological Surgeons
BMA	The British Medical Association
CEPOD	Confidential Enquiry into Perioperative Deaths
CJD	Creutzfeldt–Jakob disease
CT	Computerised Tomography
DEI	Diversity, Equality, and Inclusion
DNA	Did not arrive
DOAC	Direct Oral Anticoagulant
DRE	Digital Rectal Exam
DVT	Deep Vein Thrombosis
EMCC	European Mentoring and Coaching Council
EMG	Electromyelogram
ESWL	Extracorporeal Shock Wave Lithotripsy
FY	Foundation Year
GMC	The General Medical Council
GPs	General Practitioners
HALT	Hungry, Angry, Late, Tired
HCAs	Health Care Assistants
HIV	Human Immunodeficiency Virus
IAPOS	International Association of Physicians for the Overseas Services
ICU	Intensive Care Units
IT	Information Technology
MDU	Medical Defence Union
MPS	Medical Protection Society
MPTS	Medical Practitioners Tribunal Service
MRI	Magnetic Resonance Imaging
MRSE	Methicillin-resistant staphylococcus aureus
NEWS	National Early Warning Score
NHS	National Health Service

NHS-LA	NHS Litigation Authority
NHS-R	NHS Resolution
NPSA	National Patient Safety Agency
NTN	National Training Number
PA	Physician Assistant
PET	Positron Emission Tomography
PID	Pelvic Inflammatory Disease
PPE	Personal Protective Equipment
PSA	Prostate-Specific Antigen
RTA	Road Traffic Accident
SAS	Staff grade, associate specialist, and specialty doctors
SAU	Surgical Assessment Unit
SBAR	Situation-Background-Assessment-Recommendation
TURP	Transurethral Resection of the Prostate
UK	United Kingdom
WBAs	Web-Based Assessments
WHO	World Health Organization

Introduction to Medical Law

1

Faiz Motiwala, Hanif Motiwala,
and Sanchia S. Goonewardene

Medical law is a fascinating subject. It is one of the branches within the field of law that evokes a particularly strong response, even from a lay person. This may be in part due to the very real possibility that one may themselves require some form of healthcare in their life, but also in part due to the role of the doctor. The doctor fits the archetype of a healer, an advisor. Peculiarly, there is also a cultural sense of authority and esteem within society. The patient looks up to the doctor as a comforter or healer; one who's role is to alleviate their suffering. Nevertheless, humans retain their sense of individuality and independence. This lends itself to a unique dual relationship between a doctor and the patient. Within medicine and generally as a society, we have progressed to a stage where the is a relationship formed between the two is formed on equal ground, not a paternalistic-child role. However, doctors, while remaining one of the most highly respected professionals, are not infallible. The patient places their livelihood and well-being into the hands of the doctor whom they trust. It is natural for the public to have grown increasingly critical and expect a certain standard to be maintained.

Complaints and cases of litigation may arise from genuine malpractice, but in most cases may occur when the clinician has acted without any fault. It is commonly precipitated by an unexpected development of symptoms, delayed diagnosis or an unexpected post-operative occurrence. When the standards being met are felt

F. Motiwala
Queen Elizabeth Hospital, Woolwich, UK
e-mail: faiz.motiwala@nhs.net

H. Motiwala
Department of Urology, Southend University Hospital, Southend, UK

S. S. Goonewardene (✉)
Department of Urology, The Princess Alexandra Hospital, Harlow, UK

F. Motiwala et al. (eds.), *When Things Go Wrong In Urology*,
https://doi.org/10.1007/978-3-031-13658-0_1

to be subpar, a malpractice case can readily emerge. Not only is a malpractice case extremely destructive both to the doctor's livelihood, psychological well-being and career, it often stems from patients who feel they were wronged in their care [1]. If the care provided was suboptimal, the patient is entitled to compensation. However, although the process is daunting, it provides the opportunity for deep introspection and audit. It allows the clinician to review their practice to optimise health care delivery and reduce risk of further litigation.

By figures of NHS Resolution, the total cost of indemnity has risen drastically to £77 billion as of 31st March in 2018, from £65 billion the year prior. Total cost paid out for damages in 2017–2018 was £1.6 billion for cases of 'medical negligence', four times greater than in 2006–2007 [2, 3]. The rising rates of litigation and their associated costs may be a reflection of society and their expectations. Information is freely available and the increased level of understanding from patients regarding their conditions has precipitated our own drive towards an improved understanding, with critical appraisal and practice of evidence-based medicine.

While applicable to any specialty, this can be particularly true within the field of urology owing to the nature of the speciality. Patients may have conditions that strongly affect either their general health, the quality of their daily life, or a part of their sexuality. These can result not only in physical problems, but mental and social problems, ultimately requiring a strong holistic approach to their treatment. Among all of this, urology is an expanding speciality with planned annual increases in consultancy posts. Sub-specialities have become more defined and streamlined, ultimately leading to higher standards of care and subsequently even greater expectations of the surgeon within their field. The holistic nature of the speciality lends itself vulnerable to a barrage of medico-legal scenarios. The key to success is to learn in depth the issues surrounding medico-legal scenarios and most importantly, how to prevent these.

This book aims to highlight the common scenarios that emerge within the field of urology and provide a basis of approaching each ethical scenario the clinician may find themselves in. Included within the text are cases, some of which have gone through the court. These are utilised to illustrate aspects of good practice and highlight areas of care which could have been improved. All cases which are used are real cases, which have been summarised and anonymised where necessary. Each case will be presented with reflection regarding what went wrong and measures to protect against such measures or prevent their escalation. The cases discussed are contemporary and selected to identify those examples the reader may encounter in their practice. Some of the reflections, advice and suggestions may seem extremely obvious and basic, but have been mentioned nonetheless as a lack of these basic actions has resulted in litigation. This book does not aim to point blame or formulate discussions based purely upon hindsight. In some of these cases the surgeon has handled the case appropriately yet has unfortunately ended in litigation. Conversely, in some of the cases the surgeon has been at clear fault due to their actions (or omissions). Where relevant, the expert's opinion is included and a discussion on how we can implement this or change our practice.

1.1 A Practical Approach to Medicolegal Law

Prior to tackling scenarios and cases, we aim to lay out key concepts, basic aspects of medical law and provide an algorithm which can be applied to any case. To understand these, it is necessary to describe the basis of medical ethics laws within the UK.

Medical ethics has existed throughout history, with special obligations placed upon the doctor. Of these, the most renowned is the Hippocratic oath, with similar moral obligations existing in various cultures. These have evolved with the modern doctor requiring additional qualities including compassion, altruism, the pursuit of continuous improvement, a holistic approach and many others.

1.2 Legal Terms and Meanings

1.2.1 Medical Laws

Statutory law refers to a more formal body of the legal system; laws made in Parliament. It is mainly be based on rules and regulations mandating or prohibiting behaviours or actions of the public. In medicine it covers areas such as abortion, reproductive technology and euthanasia. It also determines the use of health data.

The human rights law is a category of statute law i.e. it is formal and non-negotiable. It contains many relevant Articles which have been relied upon to argue medical cases. The United Kingdom has incorporated the rights set out in the European Convention for the Protection of Human Rights and Fundamental Freedoms into British legislation; with the enforcement of the UK Human Right Act in 2000 [4].

Articles relevant to medical law include:

- Article 2—the right to life
- Article 3—prohibition on torture, inhuman or degrading treatment
- Article 5—the right to liberty and security
  - This protects patients against informal detention or restraint in those whom have not been sectioned
- Article 6—the right to a fair hearing or trial
- Article 8—the right to a private and family life
  - This will include elements such as a patient being able to discuss their medical problem in private, not being placed in a mixed sex ward and families being allowed to visit the patient in the hospital. It also includes elements pertaining to social care of patients at home.
- Article 9—freedom of thought, conscience and religion
- Article 10—freedom of expression
- Article 12—the right to marry and raise a family
- Article 14—securement of these rights without discrimination

1.2.2   The Common Law

The common law refers to the body of law derived from judicial decisions of court. It develops as precedents set by judges, who apply principles from previous cases and extrapolate these principles to resolve current disagreements. Judges abide by the precedents from previous cases unless the court finds a strong enough reason to challenge it or that the case is fundamentally distinct from previous cases. Cases in medicine can strongly be influenced by the common law. A well-known case will later be discussed in which the common law was critiqued and evolved.

1.2.3   Quasi-Law

Quasi (or soft) law refers to rules and guidance that are not strictly legally binding and thus do not carry legal sanctions but consist of good practice that one is expected to follow. This includes the professional guidance set out by the regulatory body of the General Medical Council (GMC), including its advice on *Good Medical Practice*. Breaches in professional conduct can lead to a multitude of sanctions including the restriction, suspension or loss of one's license to practice.

References

1. Hickey JD, Cowan J. Risk management and medicolegal issues in urology. BJU Int. 2000;86:271–4.
2. NHS Resolution presses ahead with mediation as litigation decreases but claims costs continue to rise. NHS Resolution. 2018. https://resolution.nhs.uk/2018/07/12/nhs-resolution-presses-ahead-with-mediation-as-litigation-decreases-but-claims-costs-continue-to-rise/. Accessed March 2020.
3. NHS Resolution. 2018. https://resolution.nhs.uk/wp-content/uploads/2018/09/FOI_3214_Urology.pdf. Accessed March 2020.
4. United Kingdom: Human Rights Act 1998 [United Kingdom of Great Britain and Northern Ireland], 9 November 1998.

Clinical Negligence and Malpractice

2

Faiz Motiwala, Hanif Motiwala, and Sanchia S. Goonewardene

Negligence was defined by Baron Alderson in a British case (Blyth vs Birmingham Waterworks Company) [1] in 1856:

Negligence is about causing damage to another because of a failure to exercise reasonable care; it is doing something that a reasonable person in the class of persons to which the defendant belongs would not do, or not doing something that a reasonable person in that class would do.

The defendant (Birmingham Waterworks Company) had installed a fireplug into the hydrant near Mr. Blyth's house. As the winter set in, there was a severe frost causing the plug to fail and resulting in a flood that damaged Mr. Blyth's house. Mr. Blyth then sued the company for negligence. The court found that the defendant could only have been negligent if they failed to do what a reasonable person would do in the circumstances. Severe frost could not have been in the defendant's consideration and Birmingham had not seen such cold in such time. It would therefore be unreasonable to expect the company to anticipate such an occurrence.

This principle can similarly be applied to the clinical setting i.e. providing the care that a reasonable clinician would be expected to, not an *exceptional* clinician. Making a wrong decision or incurring a bad outcome is not in itself negligent. Similarly, a junior doctor or GP will not be judged by the standards expected of a trained urologist. An act or omission may not be deemed negligent when done by

F. Motiwala
Queen Elizabeth Hospital, Woolwich, UK
e-mail: faiz.motiwala@nhs.net

H. Motiwala
Department of Urology, Southend University Hospital, Southend, UK

S. S. Goonewardene (✉)
Department of Urology, The Princess Alexandra Hospital, Harlow, UK

F. Motiwala et al. (eds.), *When Things Go Wrong In Urology*,
https://doi.org/10.1007/978-3-031-13658-0_2

the junior most member of the team but may be deemed negligent if performed by a consultant. A large element of avoiding this comes from recognising the limits of one's knowledge and abilities and being able to call on their senior or other specialty before wading into uncharted territory.

Further to this, if it can be shown in relation to a particular action or omission, that the clinician has acted "in accordance with a responsible body of medical opinion", of which the opinion had a "logical basis", then they would not be deemed negligent i.e. the Bolam test (with the Bolitho modification) [2, 3]. With respect to consent and advice however, the Montgomery ruling (discussed later) applies.

Malpractice is a subgroup of negligence and consists of four aspects. These four aspects must be proven for a patient to make a successful claim of negligence [4].

1. The duty of the healthcare professional to the patient
    *   This commences upon accepting an individual as a patient. It also occurs upon accepting to examine or treat a patient, or when a doctor agrees to be on-call and reviews a patient. This does not include when a doctor sees a patient as a non-professional in a social setting; no duty of care would be owed in this circumstance.
2. The breach of that duty
    *   This means the breach of a professional duty, to a standard of care the which a reasonable similar professional would be expected to provide to the patient. Alternatively, it may arise from an act of omission (not performing an action that would be expected of them). This may mean that expert testimony is essential unless the breach of care is obvious.
3. Injury caused by that breach/Causation issue
    *   Within the legal framework, the breach of this duty must cause some injury to the patient i.e., there must be proven injury directly linked to the clinician's misconduct. The patient may instead show a legally sufficient relationship between the injury and breach of duty, which is instead referred to proximate causation.
4. Resulting damages
    *   A claim culminates with the calculation of damages. For the purposes of reimbursement as monetary damages are easiest to calculate and administer, courts will award money damages to compensate the injured patient. These are awarded in a case to reflect the 'pain, suffering and loss of amenity' suffered as a result of the breach of duty. The values are highly variable and aim to reflect harm/damages caused to the patient; those with permanent or serious disabilities/effects may receive very large awards.

An important point to note is that the 'standard of proof' required for cases differs between criminal cases and civil cases such as these. In these cases, evidence of 51% or greater is required in favour of a particular judgement i.e., more probable than not, as opposed to criminal cases which require proof beyond reasonable doubt.

There are typically three types of patients claiming medical negligence.

1. Those genuinely harmed due to clinical negligence or poor communication
2. Those who believe something has gone wrong due to the incompetence or error of a doctor but is in reality a progression of their condition or a recognised complication of their procedure.
3. Those intending to cause disturbance for the sake of personal gain

Fortunately, the third type is rare particularly in the UK but is nonetheless a subset of patients forming claims.

Within the United Kingdom (UK), claims made against the National Health Service (NHS) are represented by the NHS Resolution (NHS-R), previously the NHS Litigation Authority (NHS LA). Fewer than 2% of the cases handled by the NHS-R reach court; these are often settled out of court or dropped by the claimant (with most ending judgement in favour of the NHS) [5].

2.1 Litigation in Urology

An analysis published in 2010 in the BJUI by Osman N. and Collins G. studied successful claims of litigation in the NHS between 1995–2009 [6]. It identified a total of 493 cases; the most common classification of claims was non-operative (232), followed by post-operative events (168) and then intraoperative events (92). The most common non-operative claim was failure to diagnose/treat cancer (69), most common intra-operative claim was perforation/organ injury (38) and most common post-operative claim was forgotten ureteric stent (23). A significant proportion of non-operative claims related to consent (24) and failure to diagnose/treat testicular torsion (21).

The most commonly implicated operative procedures were:

1. ureteroscopy/ureteric stenting (45)
2. transurethral resection of the prostate (30)
3. nephrectomy (26)
4. vasectomy (19)
5. urethral catherization (15)

What should also be noted is that while this number may seem low for a period of 14 years, it only represents successful claims. It does not encompass other patients with poor outcomes who did not pursue litigation. It also does not include all sources of urological mishap; there will be non-urological specialists e.g. obstetrics and gynaecology, spinal surgery or general surgery with urological complications.

The MDU have published their own experiences of litigation in urology over a ten-year period, and found the following common reasons for claims [7]:

- poor outcomes/complications after surgery (commonest in order being infection, renal damage, incontinence and erectile dysfunction)
- delayed diagnosis of cancer
- failure to obtain consent

The most common implicated procedures were prostatectomies, circumcisions, removal of renal stones and gender reassignment surgery. They also found that over 75% of the claims were defended however the cost of those not defended was significant, with over half of the cases costing over £100,000 each to settle, with the largest being over £2 million in compensation and legal costs (Figs. 2.1 and 2.2).

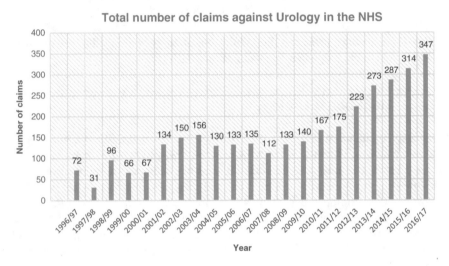

Fig. 2.1 A graphical representation of the total number of claims against Urology in the NHS between 1996–2017 [8]

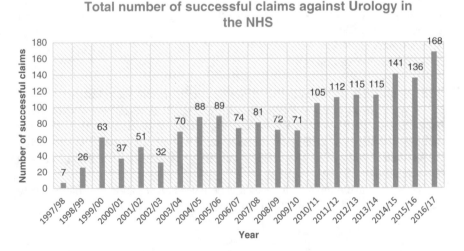

Fig. 2.2 Total number of successful claims against Urology in the NHS, between 1997–2017 [8]

Figures of NHS-R have shown an increase in both the number of both claims and number of successful claims relating to urology in the past few years, with annual rates having doubled within the last 10 years [8].

2.2   Professionalism

The General Medical Council outline several aspects expected of a doctor [9]. It reflects the core principles of being a doctor and consists of a set of values, behaviours and relationships expected. Health professionals are required to remain honest and act with integrity. This honesty relies on a certain transparency that exists beyond telling the truth, including not withholding information or deceiving a patient. This can be especially tricky when placed in scenarios of providing bad news or prognoses to patients without providing false hope (Fig. 2.3).

<u>**GMC duties of a doctor**</u>

Domain 1: Knowledge, skills and performance

- Make the care of your patient your first concern.
- Provide a good standard of practice and care.
    - Keep your professional knowledge and skills up to date.
    - Recognise and work within the limits of your competence.

Domain 2: Safety and quality

- Take prompt action if you think that patient safety, dignity or comfort is being compromised.
- Protect and promote the health of patients and the public.

Domain 3: Communication, partnership and teamwork

- Treat patients as individuals and respect their dignity.
    - Treatpatients politely and considerately.
    - Respect patients' right to confidentiality.
- Work in partnership with patients.
    - Listen to, and respond to, their concerns and preferences.
    - Give patients the information they want or need in a way they can understand.
    - Respect patients' right to reach decisions with you about their treatment and care.
    - Support patients in caring for themselves to improve and maintain their health.
- Work with colleagues in the ways that best serve patients' interests.

Domain 4: Maintaining trust

- Be honest and open and act with integrity.
- Never discriminate unfairly against patients or colleagues.
- Never abuse your patients' trust in you or the public's trust in the profession.

Fig. 2.3   GMC duties of a doctor [9]

2.3   Patient Rights

In balance with the duties expected of a doctor, it is important to consider the patient's rights. These are derived from both medical law and ethics.

- Autonomy—this consists of the ability to think, decide and act for oneself. When mental capacity is present their decisions should be respected provided there is no adverse effect on others. As such they maintain the right to accept or refuse options and ultimately make decisions which may seem irrational or harmful for them (provided it is not against the law or harmful to others)
- Justice (fairness and equity)—while the individual is the focus of daily interactions, the professional must consider the greater picture and whether the accommodation of one's wishes may deprive another. This extends even further to *distributive justice* when communal resources are scarce. There is also the *sufficiency* argument in that all individuals receive that which is essential, but opinions on what is essential vary. Fairness has to be balanced with any conflicts of interest and doctor's professional judgements not being hampered by any other factors which could include financial gain.
- Beneficence and non-maleficence (harm vs. benefit)—the provision of healthcare with the intent of doing good for the patient, while avoiding harming them or others in society. This can be tricky particularly in the evolution of modern healthcare, where actions are now deemed harmful if the person experiencing them believes it to be so or rejects them. There can be huge variety in the interpretation of this in many cases with application of common or quasi law.
- Confidentiality and public interest—patients are entitled to confidentiality in all formats of data recording. This right however is not absolute, particularly if others are at risk of harm or if there is an overriding public interest, despite the patient's wishes. Public interest is defined by law. However, care should be taken as some cases can be scrutinised as to how genuinely the public interest is at stake. This is also a principle which tends to evolve as notions of public interest change over time and technology continues to advance.
- Mental Capacity—to exercise autonomy patients require the mental capacity. This consists of being able to understand the information being conveyed, weigh up the options to come to a decision and be able to convey that decision. It is assumed unless there are grounds to make one thing otherwise, irrespective of how irrational the decision is.

References

1. England and Wales High Court (Exchequer Court) Decisions: Blyth v The Company of Proprietors of The Birmingham Waterworks. (1856). 11 Exch 781, [1856] EWHC Exch J65, 156 ER 1047.
2. Bolam v Friern Hospital Management Committee (1957). 1 WLR 583

3. Bolitho v. City and Hackney Health Authority [1996.] 4 All ER 771
4. Gittler GJ, Goldstein EJ. The elements of medical malpractice: an overview. Clin Infect Dis. 1996;23:1152–5.
5. NHS Resolution: Claims Management. https://resolution.nhs.uk/services/claims-management/. Accessed April 2020.
6. Osman N, Collins G. Urological litigation in the UK National Health Service (NHS): an analysis of 14 years of successful claims. BJU Int. 2011;108(2):162–5.
7. Learning lessons from urology claims—The MDU. https://www.themdu.com/guidance-and-advice/guides/learning-lessons-from-urology-claims. Accessed March 2020.
8. NHS Resolution. 2018. https://resolution.nhs.uk/wp-content/uploads/2018/09/FOI_3214_Urology.pdf. Accessed March 2020.
9. General Medical Council. The duties of a doctor registered with the General Medical Council. March 2013. www.gmc-uk.org/guidance/good_medical_practice/duties_of_a_doctor.asp. Accessed March 2020.

Medicolegal Pitfalls

3

Faiz Motiwala, Hanif Motiwala,
and Sanchia S. Goonewardene

3.1 An Approach to the Ethical Problem

The law and guidelines tend to provide a framework for medical practice. In some situations, two or more options would be deemed legally permissible. The challenge arises in analysing these cases and choosing the best option. This is compounded by the need to apply general principles of ethics and law to judge which elements should take precedence. Decisions should also account for all patient rights, duties of a doctor, conflict of interest, advantages/disadvantages, a balance of risk vs. benefit, in addition to the views and interests of all involved parties.

The British Medical Association (BMA) have formed an algorithm and methodology for approaching such dilemmas [1]. While some cases have clear law or can be resolved quickly by reference to GMC guidance, more complex cases require such an approach (Fig. 3.1).

The initial step is recognition of the situation and the development of an ethical issue. This may not be as obvious as one may think. For example, the provision of a new ground-breaking treatment relies not only on the clinical need of the patient and their rights, but also consideration of health equity and fairness to all. Does the provision of such a treatment deprive others of the opportunity to access other forms

F. Motiwala
Queen Elizabeth Hospital, Woolwich, UK
e-mail: faiz.motiwala@nhs.net

H. Motiwala
Department of Urology, Southend University Hospital, Southend, UK

S. S. Goonewardene (✉)
Department of Urology, The Princess Alexandra Hospital, Harlow, UK

© The Author(s), under exclusive license to Springer Nature Switzerland AG 2022
F. Motiwala et al. (eds.), *When Things Go Wrong In Urology*,
https://doi.org/10.1007/978-3-031-13658-0_3

13

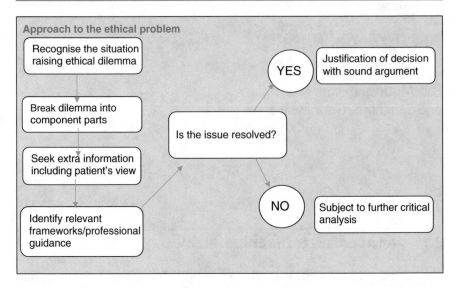

Fig. 3.1 Adapted from BMA's approach to the ethical problem

of healthcare? What determines this case to warrant this treatment over others? An ethical dilemma can emerge when the general principles one would rely upon fall short of being relevant, with multiple options.

Following this requires breaking the dilemma into components. The context and individual circumstances of each relevant party should be considered. Following this, excess detail can cloud judgement and these need to be cleared to identify key issues.

Once the crux of the situation is identified, it may reveal a lack of information in aspects of the situation. For the majority of situations, assumptions are made as to events that have occurred. An example may be that a patient complains that they were not made aware of their investigation results in due time—but what was the investigation? How long were they made to wait? Was the margin they were made to wait acceptable for their clinical state and condition? Not all of this information may be readily available. When the relevant information is reviewed, it may become apparent that the claim has no ground or merit; or conversely it may raise more concern or questions warranting further investigation.

Analysis of the dilemma also requires identification of relevant legal or professional guidance pertaining to the case. This may consist of analysing statute or common law, guidance from organisations providing medical indemnity such as the MDU or MPS, or guidance from a regulatory body such as the GMC or professional body such as the BMA.

If following this guidance, the issue has been resolved, one can simply justify their reasoning with sound argument. If it is not resolved, the issue needs further critical analysis and may in fact be necessary to seek a court declaration.

3.2   The Patient Pathway

There are several points within the patient pathway in which a clinician may find themselves attracting a litigation case. This pathway begins with the receipt of a referral letter or post-take review of a patient on the ward and continues until either discharge or review in the outpatient clinic.

In this chapter we shall highlight common pitfalls at each stage of the patient pathway; some of these are discussed in more detail in their relevant chapters.

Common pitfalls:

- History taking and examination
- Chaperones
- Diagnostics
- The Multi-disciplinary meeting
- The operation
- The post-operative period

3.2.1   History Taking and Examination

This remains the mainstay of diagnosis despite the use of various investigative modalities. Carefully taking the time to listen to patients and examining them thoroughly is critical in identification of the problem at hand. This also aids in facilitating good patient rapport for the potential long-term care required for the patient.

Examinations should always be performed and the results documented, irrespective of negative findings. There may be an unexpected finding warranting further investigation, or progression of the patient's condition on any future visits. One cannot expect to remember every single patient and there is no proof of examination without this documentation. Occasionally patients can claim the doctor did not examine them or claim an abnormality was present but was not detected. In these situations, documentation serves as proof. Lastly, although not as important as the reasons stipulated above, the examination does further the rapport with patients and provides them the notion that their concerns are not simply being dismissed.

3.2.2   Chaperones

Allegations of indecent assault can be made from male and female patients against male and female doctors. The most common is from female patients against male doctors but this does not exclude the other combinations or same sex allegations from being made.

Chaperones came into focus following the Ayling Report published in 2004 [2]. Clifford Ayling, a GP from Kent was convicted for 13 counts of indecent assault on female patients between 1991 and 1998. He was imprisoned for 4 years in December

2000 and removed from the GMC medical register in June 2001. The report was published with a number of recommendations to prevent a similar situation from occurring again.

It is highly recommended for there to be a chaperone present for examinations [3]. This is especially so for **intimate examinations** and for these they *must be* offered to the patient. You are obliged by the GMC to offer a chaperone for intimate examinations, irrespective of the gender of the patient [4]. The chaperone should be a member of the clinical team who is suitably qualified. Family members or relatives are not suitable individuals, due to the risk of inadvertent breaches of confidentiality and that if a claim was filed, they would likely side with the patient. The chaperone's name and role should also be documented in the patient notes. If a complaint arises at a future date, it is unlikely one would remember who the chaperone was. Intimate examinations include those of the breast, perineum, rectum and genitalia. It is however not only limited to these, as a patient's perception of intimate may differ from the clinician's perspective of 'routine' examination, with differences existing between various cultures as well.

Chaperones should also be offered in examining the same-sex patient. There has been a case when a female GP received a complaint from a patient who said she was touched inappropriately and that the GP had put her arm around her when examining her breasts. The complaint was withdrawn but not prior to months of stress for the doctor.

All examinations should be clearly communicated to the patient and permission sought prior to performing them. They require an explanation as to what will be performed and why it is being done. Within urology, digital rectal examinations, pelvic examinations and testicular examinations are common. Those with special interest in neurological problems may even perform the bulbocavernous reflex (for testing the acral reflex arc, nerve roots S2–S4)—elicited by squeezing the glans penis with a finger in the rectum, with an intact arc confirmed by contraction of the anus when the glans penis is squeezed. Naturally, one might assume it is a good idea both to explain to the patient what is being done and have a chaperone present during this procedure.

The chaperone should only be present for the examination itself to avoid breaches of confidentiality. With their presence it is important to remain cautious and one should wait for them to leave prior to discussing the patient's care. The chaperone's role is not complete at the end of the examination; make sure that the patient is fully dressed before allowing them to leave the room.

While a chaperone is recommended, it may not always be possible to get one. If a suitable chaperone is not available, the GMC recommend that this should be explained to the patient and if possible, offer to delay the examination. Additionally, it is a patient's right to decline a chaperone, often because they feel it is unnecessary or due to embarrassment at the involvement of a third party. They should not feel obligated to accept a chaperone. Typically, if a patient declines the chaperone most clinicians will still proceed to examination. If however you are not comfortable in proceeding without a chaperone, this should be explained to the patient and discussed with them to change their mind. If they do decline nonetheless and you remain uncomfortable, we would advise deferral of the examination to a later date. The GMC also suggest referral to another doctor though this can be inappropriate depending on the circumstances.

One should not be bound by the shackles of defensive medicine. A chaperone does not provide guarantee of protection against litigation. Someone with a chaperone may still receive a complaint, whereas the one without a chaperone may receive none.

3.2.3 Diagnostics

A significant portion of urology relies upon diagnostic investigations. These follow on from the history and examination. Most investigations are covered within national guidelines and are up to date. If an unusual investigation is required, one should not shy away and be prepared to justify them. These should however fall within the capability of the department.

Local policies will vary among NHS trusts and the consultant should be prepared to personally discuss with the radiology department should it be required. Some trusts even require a consultant-to-consultant referral for radiology investigations out of hours. While this may seem tedious it is ultimately for optimal patient care.

Beware of defensive medicine; unnecessary investigations should be avoided entirely as one can fall into the trap of over-investigation. All relevant results should be available, reviewed and acted upon as soon as possible. The responsibility of the results falls to the consultant, irrespective of the presence of a report, or if the requesting clinician was the junior. Later in this book we discuss a case with this exact issue, complicated both by over-investigation, poor follow-up and consequent unnecessary operation. Investigations should be duly followed up by the requesting clinician. Juniors should be encouraged to take responsibility of following up investigations that were requested, and consultants should be informed of any investigations that have been requested, especially if the patient is discharged with pending results. If the patient is discharged from the ward there should be a clear follow-up of results indicated in the plan.

3.2.4 The Multi-disciplinary Meeting

The advent of these meetings has been progressive in the management of uro-oncological conditions. With the presence of surgeons, oncologists and radiologists, complex cases can be discussed with optimal management plans made. Healthy arguments and discussions can also be productive and conducive for maintaining high quality standards of care (provided the environment remains healthy!).

One should not feel embarrassed to also raise less complex cases for discussion in these settings. It is better to seek a second or more colleagues' opinions on the management of these patients. Furthermore, group decisions are more likely to provide stronger defence when the management plan is questioned. The discussions and plan should be thoroughly documented including a record of who was present.

3.2.5 The Operation

The bulk of this will be covered in the chapters to come, including consent and problems in the operating theatre. The pertinent points to note include:

- It is not uncommon for the patient who is seen in clinic to be operated on by a different surgeon. In these cases, clear documentation and communication between team members is essential for good continuity of care.
- Provide patients with BAUS procedure leaflets to aid in the consent process.
- Check the notes, consent and images are correct prior and meet the patient prior to their being anaesthetised (including orientation of images!). Verify these with the patient. This requires one to be organised and punctual. Patients should be marked, and this should be clear and unambiguous. Some surgeons have also adopted adding the operation, or signature and date next to the marking.
- If there are concerns do not let the anaesthetist prevent you from disturbing the patient in the anaesthetic room (this has been identified as a factor contributing to a potential error!)
- Patient identification—Do not gloss over the briefing and other aspects of the 'Five steps to safer surgery'. A failure here can result in a failure of multiple steps beyond the basic wrong site/surgery, including appropriate deep vein thrombosis (DVT) or antibiotic prophylaxis.
- The surgeon should be satisfied with the planned operation, side and site prior to draping of the patient.
- Inappropriate delegation—although rarer in this era, it is important to ensure the junior surgeon can perform the planned operation. There have been incidents where this was not the case, resulting in post-operative complications and legal actions being filed. As a junior, you should not feel pressured or unable to ask for help, and as the consultant, should ensure they know you are happy to come in and assist. If this is not possible, ensure that a named consultant colleague is available and happy to provide cover. This is not to dissuade independence from junior surgeons, but to remain sensible about what one can do as this will significantly vary dependant on their experiences and seniority. A more extreme view is to simply not delegate to juniors which reduces the risk of litigation and is already adopted by some surgeons. However, this is not ideal for training of future surgeons and may limit what one can accomplish in a given time period.

3.2.6 The Post-operative Period

It is good practice to see your own patients following an operation, clearly documenting your review and plan. Patients are appreciative of you coming to see them when they have woken up in recovery, and there is far less a likelihood of any miscommunication for their follow-up. Daily ward round reviews should occur and this should be documented. It is rarer these days though not uncommon for there to be 'no review' of a patient on a particular day (which may simply be a lack of documentation), or review by only the junior most team member. Ideally ward rounds should be led by consultants or at the very least a consultant board round should occur; in some areas this is a practice already adopted.

The ward round entries should be relevant and encompass the information required. Essential elements include the date and time, who was leading or present in the round, the patient's general status, current trend, relevant investigations, observations, urine output, drain or nephrostomy output, relevant examination findings such as the status of their abdomen, wound or dressing, and a clear plan for the day.

In some cases there may be several patients requiring shared care with Urology e.g. with Medicine, General Surgery, Obstetrics and Gynaecology etc. There is the potential for miscommunication and difficulty in co-ordinating care as these patients may lack a lead clinician. The team needs to be mindful of seeing their patient and not being dismissive of any issues noted, incorrectly believing the other team will resolve the issue at hand unless. There should be a clear primary responsible clinician and clear delegation of who will perform particular tasks.

It is also essential for juniors to be taught the adequate skill and expertise, with a system of communication should the need for escalation arise. They should be aware of the pertinent aspects to observe for in the post-operative period and be able to recognise the deteriorating patient. General training and courses are now performed such that these requirements should be met, however in-house training may also be required as additional support, or for specifics such as identifying the signs and symptoms of bladder perforation, or the management of post-operative haematuria. The required knowledge should be highlighted at induction for new members to the department, including educating the team with written guidelines or handbooks surmising pre- and post-operative care, trust policies and things to be aware of. Even better would be to hold teaching sessions that cover these aspects. It is unreasonable to expect optimal care and excellent outcomes if adequate education is not given to those providing the care on the wards!

References

1. Medical Ethics Today. The BMA's handbook of ethics and law. Germany: Wiley; 2012.
2. Ayling Report Committee of inquiry independent investigation into how the NHS handled allegation about the conduct of Clifford Ayling. 2004. http://www.dh.gov.uk/asset-Root/04/08/90/65/04089065.pdf. Accessed March 2020
3. Richardson C. Chaperones: who needs them? BMJ. 2005;330:s17.
4. Intimate examinations and chaperones (summary). General Medical Council. https://www.gmc-uk.org/ethical-guidance/ethical-guidance-for-doctors/intimate-examinations-and-chaperones. Accessed May 2020

Communication in Healthcare

4

Faiz Motiwala, Hanif Motiwala,
and Sanchia S. Goonewardene

Communication is at the heart of legal complaints. Often the first hurdle and pitfall for many doctors is how they communicate with their patients; when done well it allows the establishment of good rapport. When done poorly it can lead to series of outcomes ranging from a slight confusion or misunderstanding, to a barrage of complaints [1]. It is very much a clinical skill and the application of it can determine good clinical practice and patient satisfaction. The GMC stress its importance [2] and many medical schools have increasingly introduced it as a clinical skill to learn and cultivate from the beginning of medical school. The importance of this communication extends to communicating with other staff members such as ward clerks, therapists, nurses, HCAs as well as between doctors on the same clinical team or between different specialties.

4.1   Discussions with Patients

The most common themes in complaints suggest that patients are more likely to resort to medico-legal consultation when there is a breakdown in communication. These may arise from difficulty in contacting the clinician, if the patient is met with a defensive, arrogant or condescending attitude, or being provided an inadequate

F. Motiwala
Queen Elizabeth Hospital, Woolwich, UK
e-mail: faiz.motiwala@nhs.net

H. Motiwala
Department of Urology, Southend University Hospital, Southend, UK

S. S. Goonewardene (✉)
Department of Urology, The Princess Alexandra Hospital, Harlow, UK

© The Author(s), under exclusive license to Springer Nature
Switzerland AG 2022
F. Motiwala et al. (eds.), *When Things Go Wrong In Urology*,
https://doi.org/10.1007/978-3-031-13658-0_4

explanation from the clinician [3]. The importance of communication cannot be emphasised more. In these circumstances the clinician should place themselves in the patient's position and attempt to understand their situation. By embracing the situation, it enables the clinician to clear any misunderstandings, work to resolve the situation and prevent recurrences in the future.

Within urology many of the patients' conditions are a sensitive topic and procedures have known complications associated with them that can continue to impact quality of life. It is imperative that the patient has a full understanding of their condition and a realistic expectation is provided.

Speak in simple terms, avoid use of technical jargon—peeing instead of micturition, bleeding instead of haemorrhage. Vivid descriptions and colourful language have their place but may not be the most sensible choice in a discussion with patients (or in clinical records for that matter). Care should be taken when describing the course of events in an operation and particularly in the use of technical jargon. While it may prove one's intellect and increase a patient's respect for you, some will not understand what you are saying rendering the conversation relatively pointless. More importantly one should note whether the patient is absorbing the information being presented to them. Are they deaf? Are they just nodding along? Is English their first language or is an interpreter necessary?

One should also attribute due caution to describing events to patients. The patient may interpret or latch onto terms such as, 'a lot of pulling' or 'sudden haemorrhage'. To the surgeon these can be of little concern but to the lay person may suggest something terrible has happened to them; the term 'haemorrhage' in and of itself suggests a more serious connotation than the term 'bleeding' in the colloquial language. Careless remarks easily roll off the tongue and have been highlighted in reports, such as when a bereaved daughter was told "death is rarely an ideal situation for anyone" and that "truth be told your mother probably said her goodbyes long before the final moments" [3]. Needless to say, the daughter did not respond well to the remark.

Unless you have a good long-standing relationship with a patient or the atmosphere is appropriate, you should generally avoid laughing or cracking jokes during the consultation. Laughing can be viewed as inappropriate or offensive to some patients. An amusing joke may lose its hilarity when it is being repeated back to you in the court by the claimant's lawyer. That is not to say you should remain stone-faced and unflinching during the consultation. Consultations are not just about seeking information; they form and establish rapport for a presumably long relationship that they might trust your judgement. It is not beyond a surgeon to be friendly and sociable!

Another facet to communication is the body language depicted to the patient. Communication is a duality; it does not consist only of speaking. Take the time to listen attentively to your patients, show empathy and an expression of understanding of their concerns. Simple mannerisms include turning your body toward the patient and giving them due attention; at that moment in time they should feel that they are the most important person to you. Watching the clock, paying attention to your bleep or being distracted by minor things are not the recommend ways to instil confidence and trustworthiness in your patient.

Be clear in the words used to describe something. Often this stems from discomfort in telling a patient out of the fear of upsetting them. For example, terms such as 'growth' have been used to describe cancer which can be interpreted in a multitude of ways. Using unclear terms can cause confusion or cause a patient to lose confidence or trust in their clinician. The worst consequence of this that it can lull people into a false sense of security. This can result in their failure to keep important appointments or chase results if there is a breakdown in administrative follow-up which can become a brewing complaint or worse. While one's compassion may drive them to use euphemisms or avoid clear terms, these should only be reserved for when there is genuine concern that using clear terms would be detrimental to their health or care. Otherwise be clear. If you mean 'cancer', say 'cancer'.

In these circumstances, one may not be simply suggesting the possible diagnosis, but rather telling them a diagnosis. "Breaking bad news" is a common requirement for any doctor. It is a complex and sensitive task, requiring a compassionate and tactful approach. The right approach can make coping with a difficult situation easier for a patient and their family. In 2000, Baile and colleagues published in The Oncologist a six-step model for disclosing this information—the widely popularised SPIKES model (Fig. 4.1) [4].

SPIKES

- **Set up**
  - Plan the discussion in advance. Choose an appropriate quiet location with enough seating.
  - Suggest to the patient to be accompanied by a significant other.
  - Put your bleep on silent or give it to someone else to prevent any interruptions.
  - Establish rapport. Make a connection with the patient through means such as eye contact or holding their arm (if appropriate).
- **Perception**
  - Employ the principle "before you tell, ask." Allow the patient to express their emotions and ask questions.
  - Open ended question to establish what the patient knows and help guide the delivery of your information/message.
- **Invitation**
  - Check the patient or relatives are actually willing to listen to what you say or if they are avoiding listening to you
  - If they are avoiding details, offer to speak in the future or discuss with family / friends if appropriate

Fig. 4.1 A model of SPIKES—adapted from Baile and colleagues' publication

- **Knowledge**
    - A warning the patient of bad news can lessen the shock of its disclosure
    - Provide information at an appropriate pace
    - Use appropriate language – avoid technical jargon
    - Provide information in small chunks and check their understanding periodically.
    - Reassure the patient of ongoing support (especially with a poor prognosis!)
- **Empathy**
    - Allow a brief period to give them the time to absorb the information and express their emotions
    - Observe and validate the patient's emotions
- **Strategy and summary**
    - Make sure they understand by summarising the pertinent points and encourage them to express their concerns.
    - Provide some material for them to absorb when they are ready
    - Suggest the option to note down any information to properly address these questions at a next meeting.

Fig. 4.1 (continued)

The approach can be applied for any situation or person. You may be telling a patient that their renal cancer has recurred despite their nephrectomy or updating the patient's relatives that their loved one is fighting for their life in ICU. Discussion with family members or friends can seem a daunting task but is a common occurrence and essential in some circumstances. Friends or relatives can provide a secondary history or act as a second pair of eyes or ears. Their helpfulness should not be underestimated when explaining conditions to patients or seeking consent for procedures.

4.2   The Angry Patient

An angry patient or relative is an unavoidable truth in clinical practice. There are always reasons behind a patient's anger such as bad news, fear, or misunderstandings. They may have been kept waiting for their appointment, investigation, or treatment, they may have suffered a complication, or perhaps it is simply a culmination of all the problems in their life.

Whatever the reason may be, it is important to stay cool and calm. Never respond to an angry patient with anger, despite any temptation to raise your voice or argue with the patient. Place yourself in their shoes and try to understand what is driving their anger. Apologise for their situation. Empathise. Be patient. Be supportive. This is one of the situations where you want to use your body language to tell them they have your full attention. Legitimising their anger, for example with a phrase such as 'I understand you are upset...' shows you are paying attention to them and allows them the opportunity to explain themselves [5]. Using the term 'I understand how you feel...' may do more harm, causing them to challenge you despite your best intentions. Empathising with the patient's feelings shows them that you do care and wish for their well-being. This will work in the majority of cases with the patient viewing you as a friend as opposed to an adversary, allowing you to work towards a solution.

If despite your best attempts they continue to be angry or if physical aggression is imminent, tell them calmly and clearly that you cannot continue any further discussion with them in these circumstances. Inform them you are going to leave the room and give them the chance to cool off. Offer them a second opinion or to see your colleague at a later date, if you feel this to be the source of the problem.

It is vital to protect yourself and others in these circumstances and should call security if required. On some occasions the police may need to be involved and you would have to justify disclosing confidential information to them.

Make sure to record details of the consultation, noting what was said. Direct quotations are helpful. Record explanations provided and the apologies made. This act of writing can also help you to reflect on the situation. Speaking to angry patients can be quite taxing and you may need a break or relax before seeing the next patient to ensure you are calm and attentive. If you have the time, discussing with a trusted colleague can be helpful.

4.3 Managing Patient Expectations

From the moment a patient chooses to seek healthcare, expectations are formed in their mind consciously or subconsciously. A simple expectation may be simply for them to find out what their problem is or how to treat it. A more complex expectation may arise from the desire of a particular investigation to exclude a particular problem before a basic assessment is even performed. For each encounter, patients will have differing expectations. These expectations have shifted alongside advances in medical care, including their desire to complain should they receive care they perceive to be inadequate.

The rising number of complaints are not shown to be associated with a reduction in the quality of care provided; this is evident in claims being filed relating to non-clinical reasons such as poor communication [6, 7]. The surgeon may perceive the care they provided was good, viewing success purely from clinical outcomes. In contrast, the patient may place emphasis on the overall experience and other factors such if they felt cared for. So, for what reasons can we view the same experience differently?

4.3.1 Information

Patients can often attend appointments with a perception of their diagnosis and the treatment required. Universal access to the internet has meant patients can find information (often inaccurate) from numerous websites. They may also have been informed certain things from either the GP or A&E physicians which is contradictory to the specialist opinion. This may result in expectations of investigations or treatment that may not be offered or simply inappropriate for their symptoms. Conversely patients may have a lack of information and not expect prolonged waiting times for their appointment, or that their symptom of visible haematuria may in fact be a brewing bladder cancer.

4.3.2   Time Pressures

Perceptions of time can greatly vary. Clinicians can see 10–20 patients in a general day or clinic, whereas for that one patient that patient there is only that one appointment. The emphasis placed on an interaction can be influenced by the allotted clinic times and other commitments, such as an unwell patient or a patient requiring emergency surgery. A short or rushed encounter can make it difficult to check with a patient if they can fully understand the condition, diagnosis, reasons for investigations and treatment options. When relevant, offer leaflets and the opportunity for the patient to relay information back to you and ask questions. Seek the support of other colleagues or seniors when you are struggling in these situations, especially with the concern of quality of care being compromised. If it is a situation with a general shortage of staff, the service manager and departmental lead should be made aware.

Within the outpatient clinic setting, the view of BAUS is that enormous clinics are no longer appropriate [8]. There needs to be adequate time to provide patients with relevant information to allow them make decisions, to provide counselling, and to document the discussion surrounding the consent process. The generally suggested numbers for an outpatient clinic with new and follow-up patients is approximately 12 (6 new and 6 follow-ups, assuming 15 min for follow-up patients and 20 min for new patients). This length of time should allow for dictation of letters. Of course, these numbers will vary between each surgeon and what you are comfortable with. Patients with cancer may require even longer consultations e.g., 30 min as these may involve breaking bad news. Specialist complex clinics typically require longer clinic times with new patients requiring between 30–45 min. Other clinics such as the one stop clinic include many more investigations and a full review of the patient and as such should have more dedicated time e.g., 40–50 min. Unfortunately, these recommendations are not always followed, with some people seeing a larger number of patients and not being able to give enough time to each patient. If there are persisting issues with patient numbers in the clinic setting, a trainee should escalate to their consultant and supervisor. As a consultant, this should be escalated to the service manager, and subsequently the clinical director if required. Patient care should never be compromised.

4.3.3   Patient Anxiety or Depression

Patients may be anxious or depressed when being reviewed, compounding any of the above factors and increasing the possibility of misunderstandings arising. Although there are no clear solutions to this problem (especially when might not even be aware that the patient is anxious or depressed), you can still adopt and apply principles such as those in the SPIKES model. Being empathetic and understanding of their plight will establish a sense of rapport and meet the expectations from some patients. Remain patient. Be clear and use simple language, avoiding technical jargon. Invite them to have someone close to them involved in the discussions. Allow them to ask questions without speaking over them. On the more serious topics you may want to check they have absorbed the information by asking them to repeat it back to you. Information from clinic appointments can be supplemented with leaflets or posters in waiting rooms. If the patient is someone who explores the recesses of the internet about information on their condition, refer them to reputable websites such as the BAUS website (baus.org.uk), 'patient.co.uk' or the NHS website with the specific details of their condition.

4.4   Communicating with Staff

There should be clear active communication between the team members. In fact, a significant proportion of medical errors can be avoided through good communication and collaboration between team members. Ensure there is a clear system of communication between seniors and juniors, especially for the junior to contact the senior in case of emergency. They should not fear contacting the on-call consultant for advice on clinical or administrative problems. The team should also be mindful of the atmosphere and any discussions in front of patients, especially during procedures under local anaesthetic or cystoscopies. It can be friendly and pleasant (which is preferable!) but must remain sufficiently professional. If any of the staff laugh and joke during the procedures or in conversation about the patient, these may be misconstrued by the patient as laughter at their expense. Some of these procedures can seem minor or inconsequential to us due to the sheer number we perform but can be an uncomfortable and worrying time for the patient. It remains our responsibility to conduct ourselves with due manner and preserve the patient's dignity.

References

1. Koul PA. Effective communication, the heart of the art of medicine. Lung India. 2017;34(1):95–6.
2. General Medical Council. The duties of a doctor registered with the General Medical Council. March 2013. www.gmc-uk.org/guidance/good_medical_practice/duties_of_a_doctor.asp. Accessed March 2020.
3. UK Parliamentary and Health Service Ombudsman—Listening and Learning report. November 2012. https://www.theioi.org/ioi-news/current-news/release-of-report-listening-and-learning. Accessed May 2020.
4. Baile WF, Buckman R, Lenzi R, Glober G, Beale EA, Kudelka AP. SPIKES—A six-step protocol for delivering bad news: application to the patient with cancer. Oncologist. 2000;5(4):302–11.
5. Dingley C, Daugherty K, Derieg MK, et al. Improving patient safety through provider communication strategy enhancements. In: Henriksen K, Battles JB, Keyes MA, et al., editors. Advances in patient safety: new directions and alternative approaches (Vol. 3: Performance and tools). Rockville, MD: Agency for Healthcare Research and Quality (US); 2008.

6. O'Daniel M, Rosenstein AH. Professional communication and team collaboration (Chapter 33). In: Hughes RG, editor. Patient safety and quality: an evidence-based handbook for nurses. Rockville, MD: Agency for Healthcare Research and Quality (US); 2008.
7. Ha JF, Longnecker N. Doctor-patient communication: a review. Ochsner J. 2010;10(1):38–43.
8. A guide to job planning for consultant urologists. BAUS. 2016. https://www.baus.org.uk/_user-files/pages/files/Publications/2016%20Job%20Planning%20for%20Consultants.pdf. Accessed May 2020.

When Communication Goes Wrong in Medicine

5

Karan R. Chadda, Ellen E. Blakey,
and Sanchia S. Goonewardene

Patient-centered care is essential in the modern practice of medicine and relies on good communication amongst healthcare workers and to patients and their families. Studies have shown that when communication goes wrong, there is an increase in preventable adverse events [1, 2] and approximately 27% of malpractice is due to issues with communication [3]. Indeed, poor communication forms the basis of many NHS complaints, even more so than complaints regarding clinical competence [4, 5]. Interestingly, a previous survey showed that 75% of surgeons deemed that their communication towards their patients was satisfactory compared to only 21% of patients [6]. This shows that there is a clear mismatch to what doctors and patients perceive as a successful consultation in terms of communication.

5.1   Between the Doctor and Patient

Effective communication has been associated with increased patient satisfaction and health status [7]. Furthermore, when healthcare professionals actively listen and take the time to understand patient concerns, patients are more likely to acknowledge and comply with treatments and lifestyle changes [8, 9]. A crucial but often overlooked aspect of communication is non-verbal. For example, maintaining eye contact and acknowledging gestures shows an interest and aids history taking. With modern medicine, the increased use of technology such as consulting room computer has been associated with negative body posture, reduced eye contact and attention [10]. Added to the time constraints of clinical practice and service provision, the reduced quality of interaction results in a lack of shared decision-making.

K. R. Chadda (✉) · E. E. Blakey
Cambridge University Hospitals NHS Foundation Trust, Cambridge, UK

S. S. Goonewardene
The Princess Alexandra Hospital, Harlow, UK

Yet, it is increasingly becoming an ethical and legal requirement to involve patients in decision-making, such as obtaining consent before any procedure. This was highlighted by the Montgomery case, which applied a patient focused test to UK law by instituting a duty of care to warn patients of material risks that a reasonable person in their position would likely attach significance [11]. Obtaining consent in medicine and surgery thus clearly depends on effective communication to adequately explain the reasons behind and the benefits and risks of any procedure in a way that can be clearly understood.

5.2   Between Healthcare Professionals

It is important to acknowledge that errors in communication are not limited to doctor-patient interactions but also intra-and inter-professional communication. Studies have shown that inadequacies with processes and systems that facilitate clinical handover between doctors result in communication errors [12]. For example, hospital doctors frequently would like more detail from referral letters and general practitioners (GPs) would like more clarity in follow up plans. Indeed, a study showed that half of GPs felt like their questions were not fully addressed from the referral process [13]. Both hospital and community doctors acknowledge that service provision demands and hence lack of time is a contributing factor to the suboptimal written communication [14]. It is important to improve the process to allow for better continuity of care in the best interests of the patient.

Within hospital, efficient interprofessional communication improves satisfaction, decreases adverse events and shortens length of hospital stay, whereas ineffective communication puts patient safety at risk and wastes resources [15]. For example, in the intensive care setting, a study showed that ineffective communication between nurses and doctors resulted in up to 37% of errors [16]. A recent review summarized potential strategies to improve on inter-professional communication, which included having checklists, team training, work shift evaluation and using a SBAR (situation-background-assessment-recommendation) template [15]. In particular, the SBAR tool has been seen to increase the effectiveness of handovers in hospital [17, 18]. The tool was created to facilitate delivering salient information in a logical, concise manner that enables the receiver to have an improved understanding and give timely, correct advice [17].

5.3   Between Healthcare Professionals and Family Members

Communicating to families to collect collateral history and update them on the clinical situation are important roles of healthcare staff. It enables staff to better understand the background of the patient and gives an opportunity for relatives to have any concerns addressed. This became even more crucial during the COVID-19 pandemic when family members were unable to physically visit their loved ones in hospital and in many cases solely relied on healthcare staff updating them over the phone. Despite its clear importance, it has been shown that some families find that clinicians lack good communication skills and use medical jargon that they do not understand [19]. As opposed to ineffective communication, sometimes it is simply the lack of communication between staff and families that lead to complaints. For example, *The More Care, Less Pathway* report found a lack of communication to family that their relative was approaching end of life [4]. From a staff perspective, problems with communication have been attributed to concerns about giving false information, uncertainty regarding prognosis and the demands of service provision, with measures of efficiency not accounting for time spent updating relatives [4].

5.4   Communication Teaching

As highlighted, suboptimal communication between various groups can be cata-strophic on patient care and satisfaction. As a result, communication skills should form a pivotal role in medical education. Unfortunately, implementation in com-munication skills teaching has historically been limited. This likely stems from lim-ited evidence in teaching methods when facilitators were trained, with a focus on experiential learning. Increased experience does not necessarily result in a good facilitator. With lack of structured guidance, experiential learning can lead to bad habit formation whereby communication is compromised [20].

There are two aspects of communication. The 'content' of communication focuses on the information that needs to be gained in order to reach an appropriate differential diagnosis [21]. The traditional history taking method focuses on obtain-ing this. Also vital in communication is the 'process', which encompasses the skills (both verbal, and non-verbal), and the structure an interview must take to success-fully gain the information required. The Calgary-Cambridge methods of communi-cation revolutionized communication skills teaching. It is an easily accessible framework, based around 5 key tasks that should form the basis of any clinical encounter as outlined below [20]:

1. Initiating the session
2. Gathering information
3. Building relationship/facilitating patient's involvement
4. Explanation and planning
5. Closing the session

Kurtz et al. [21] further developed the Calgary-Cambridge method of communica-tion by focusing on the integration of 'content' and 'process'. This was achieved by developing three diagrams. These schemata are more translatable to real life, outlin-ing the use of the biomedical aspect, patient perspective, and physical examination to reach a diagnosis and enable a management plan to be discussed with the patient. The clearly structured method and breakdown of tasks and skills makes it more accessible to both facilitators and learners [21]. It allows facilitators, learners, and colleagues to identify the part of the medical interview you are in and provide systematic feedback. Regular giving and receiving of feedback subsequently improves quality of communication [22].

Teaching communication skills early in medical training increases competence, patient satisfaction and outcomes [23]. It also instills a positive attitude to communication skills training and appreciation of the importance of such. As a post-graduate trainee's clinical competence evolves, communication skills must also evolve to deal with complexity, whilst still maintaining a good doctor-patient relationship. Despite this, the skills learned in medical school can depreciate over the course of training [21]. The Calgary-Cambridge method of communication is applicable to all levels of training and therefore should be an established part of the training curriculum throughout.

5.5   Future of Communication

The method of teaching communication must be adaptable to change. The shift to more digital encounters has been more of a necessity in recent times due to COVID-19 and its associated hospital policies, shielding, and social isolation [24]. The GMC have issued guidance on when remote, online consultations are appropriate, and when face to face consultations are required. Furthermore, NICE has issued a guide on when to use, how to plan, and tips on how to carry out an online medical encounter [24].

There are some clear advantages to online consultations. It enabled ongoing access to healthcare during the COVID-19 pandemic. By having reduced face to face contact, patients have reduced exposure to transmissible diseases. The ability to undergo telephone or online consultations from home or various other settings makes online healthcare easily accessible to patients. Likely because of this, patients who frequently did not attend appointments previously were found to have increased attendance with the introduction to online consultations [25]. Digital healthcare also has a positive socio-economic impact through reducing the time and cost of travel to healthcare settings.

Additionally, with remote access, less time is needed to be taken off work [25]. Online or telephone consultations require infrastructure and software to be in place, both by the patient and the healthcare professional. By introducing digital medical encounters, healthcare inequalities could be exaggerated. Furthermore, online communication introduces challenges regarding privacy, confidentiality and ability to raise safeguarding concerns [25]. There is always a risk of breaching data through online systems and ability to carry out such consultations in various settings could compromise privacy.

Effective communication to come to a diagnosis can be compromised through the medium of telephone or video. Non-verbal cues are impossible to pick up over the phone and can be masked through video consultation. This can compromise the expression of empathy and subsequent doctor- patient relationship [26]. Additionally, physical examination normally forms a key role in diagnosis. Some examinations can be done over video, but others would not be possible. Physical examination can be done through patient self-examination or with the help of relatives or carers [27]. There is a limit on how effective examination though the video platform can be. It heavily relies upon clear communication between patient and doctor, technical aspects such as lighting, and patients' access to and operation of equipment required.

The 'NHS long term plan' (2019) outlines an aim to increase digital medical encounters [28]. One target within this plan was to reduce face to face consultations by one third within five years. Although COVID-19 has resulted in preference towards digital consultations, there remains to be significant challenges to be overcome to minimize communication errors. As with the rest of medicine, the circumstances in which communication goes wrong are likely to evolve over time and so must the ways we overcome this.

References

1. Bartlett G, Blais R, Tamblyn R, Clermont RJ, Macgibbon B. Impact of patient communication problems on the risk of preventable adverse events in acute care settings. CMAJ. 2008;178:1555–62.
2. Wilson RM, Runciman WB, Gibberd RW, Harrison BT, Newby L, Hamilton JD. The quality in Australian Health Care Study. Med J Aust. 1995;163:458–71.
3. Tiwary A, Rimal A, Paudyal B, Sigdel KR, Basnyat B. Poor communication by health care professionals may lead to life-threatening complications: examples from two case reports. Wellcome Open Res. 2019;4:7.
4. Caswell G, Pollock K, Harwood R, Porock D. Communication between family carers and health professionals about end-of-life care for older people in the acute hospital setting: a qualitative study. BMC Palliat Care. 2015;14:35.
5. Ha JF, Longnecker N. Doctor-patient communication: a review. Ochsner J. 2010;10:38–43.
6. Tongue JR, Epps HR, Forese LL. Communication skills for patient-centered care: research-based, easily learned techniques for medical interviews that benefit orthopaedic surgeons and their patients. JBJS. 2005;87:652–8.
7. Ong LM, De Haes JC, Hoos AM, Lammes FB. Doctor-patient communication: a review of the literature. Soc Sci Med. 1995;40:903–18.
8. Stewart, M. A. Effective physician-patient communication and health outcomes: a review. CMAJ. 1995;152:1423–33.
9. Street, R. L., Jr. How clinician-patient communication contributes to health improvement: modeling pathways from talk to outcome. Patient Educ Couns. 2013;92:286–91.
10. Noordman J, Verhaak P, Van Beljouw I, Van Dulmen S. Consulting room computers and their effect on general practitioner–patient communication. Family Practice. 2010;27:644–51.
11. Chan SW, Tulloch E, Cooper ES, Smith A, Wojcik W, Norman JE. Montgomery and informed consent: where are we now? BMJ. 2017;357:j2224.
12. Campbell P, Torrens C, Pollock A, Maxwell M. A scoping review of evidence relating to communication failures that lead to patient harm. https://www.gmc-uk.org/-/media/documents/a-scoping-review-of-evidence-relating-to-communication-failures-thatlead-to-patient-harm_p-80569509.pdf.
13. Vermeir P, Vandijck D, Degroote S, Peleman R, Verhaeghe R, Mortier E, Hallaert G, Van Daele S, Buylaert W, Vogelaers D. Communication in healthcare: a narrative review of the literature and practical recommendations. Int J Clin Pract. 2015;69:1257–67.
14. Gandhi TK, Sittig DF, Franklin M, Sussman AJ, Fairchild DG, Bates DW. Communication breakdown in the outpatient referral process. J Gen Intern Med. 2000;15:626–31.

15. Wang YY, Wan QQ, Lin F, Zhou WJ, Shang SM. Interventions to improve communication between nurses and physicians in the intensive care unit: an integrative literature review. Int J Nurs Sci. 2018;5:81–8.
16. Donchin Y, Gopher D, Olin M, Badihi Y, Biesky M, Sprung CL, Pizov R, Cotev S. A look into the nature and causes of human errors in the intensive care unit. Crit Care Med. 1995;23:294–300.
17. De Meester K, Verspuy M, Monsieurs KG, Van Bogaert P. SBAR improves nurse-physician communication and reduces unexpected death: a pre and post intervention study. Resuscitation. 2013;84:1192–6.
18. Joffe E, Turley JP, Hwang KO, Johnson TR, Johnson CW, Bernstam EV. Evaluation of a problem-specific SBAR tool to improve after-hours nurse-physician phone communication: a randomized trial. Jt Comm J Qual Patient Saf. 2013;39:495–501.
19. Robinson J, Gott M, Ingleton C. Patient and family experiences of palliative care in hospital: what do we know? An integrative review. Palliat Med. 2014;28:18–33.
20. Kurtz SM, Silverman JD. The Calgary-Cambridge Referenced Observation Guides: an aid to defining the curriculum and organizing the teaching in communication training programmes. Med Educ. 1996;30:83–9.
21. Kurtz S, Silverman J, Benson J, Draper J. Marrying content and process in clinical method teaching: enhancing the Calgary-Cambridge guides. Acad Med. 2003;78:802–9.
22. Maguire P, Fairbairn S, Fletcher C. Consultation skills of young doctors: I—Benefits of feedback training in interviewing as students persist. Br Med J (Clin Res Ed). 1986;292:1573–6.
23. Choudhary A, Gupta V. Teaching communications skills to medical students: Introducing the fine art of medical practice. Int J Appl Basic Med Res. 2015;5:S41–4.
24. England N, Improvement N. Clinical guide for the management of remote consultations and remote working in secondary care during the coronavirus pandemic. NHSE. 2020;
25. Quinn LM, Davies MJ, Hadjiconstantinou M. Virtual consultations and the role of technology during the COVID-19 pandemic for people with Type 2 diabetes: the UK perspective. J Med Internet Res. 2020;22:e21609.
26. Liu X, Sawada Y, Takizawa T, Sato H, Sato M, Sakamoto H, Utsugi T, Sato K, Sumino H, Okamura S, Sakamaki T. Doctor-patient communication: a comparison between telemedicine consultation and face-to-face consultation. Intern Med. 2007;46:227–32.
27. Car J, Koh GC, Foong PS, Wang CJ. Video consultations in primary and specialist care during the covid-19 pandemic and beyond. BMJ. 2020;371:m3945.
28. England N, Improvement N. Clinical guide for the management of remote consultations and remote working in secondary care during the coronavirus pandemic. NHSE. 2020.

Communication Between Different Levels Within a Team

6

Sanchia S. Goonewardene, Hanif Motiwala, and Faiz Motiwala

Discussion between seniors and juniors at all levels can sometimes be something very difficult. It is important as a junior doctor, that your seniors understand all points of patient care when you are speaking to them. This is in line with Good Medical Practice, Duties of a Doctor. It is vital that all information is put forward in a structured way, so it is easily understandable.

6.1 Tools Available for Communication

There are a variety of tools available to communicate pieces of information in bite sized pieces. One of these tools, is SBAR. Situation-Background-Assessment-Recommendation. This allows you to maintain focus, provides clarity to your words, and helps to give a structured approach to any patient information you convey.

6.2 Prevention of Medical Errors

There are two simple measures that really help prevent medical errors: thinking one step ahead of the game and informing your seniors. As a junior registrar, approximately 6 h each week are spent preparing lists; from checking urines, to reviewing

S. S. Goonewardene (✉)
Department of Urology, The Princess Alexandra Hospital, Harlow, UK

H. Motiwala
Department of Urology, Southend University Hospital, Southend, UK

F. Motiwala
Queen Elizabeth Hospital, Woolwich, UK
e-mail: faiz.motiwala@nhs.net

© The Author(s), under exclusive license to Springer Nature Switzerland AG 2022
F. Motiwala et al. (eds.), *When Things Go Wrong In Urology*,
https://doi.org/10.1007/978-3-031-13658-0_6

35

scans and phoning patients. On one occasion a patient was listed for a distal ureteric stone extraction. The CT scan was out of date, so I liaised with the radiology department and with their help, the patient was scanned a week before his operation. The CT scan demonstrated he had passed the distal ureteric stone and a 'never event' was prevented as a result. The lesson is to always prepare your lists 2 weeks in advance—it gives you time to scan. Spend the time to do this in detail and inform your seniors of the outcome results.

6.3   Know When You Are Out of Your Depth

The other key factor in being a junior and managing your seniors, is to recognise when you are out of your depth and know who to contact, with a back-up plan in mind. As a junior registrar, I had worked in a Trust very often without a consultant on-site. During the second day of my first week on call, I had a patient that required an emergency case to stent in theatre. As a courtesy, I rang the consultant on call to let him know what I was doing. He was not on site. After quickly ringing around, I learnt that all consultants were off-site or on leave. There were no senior middle grades available. The most senior person available was an ST5. I was taking the stent to theatre, but I was on my own. The case was taken to theatre by myself and stented. Thankfully it was straightforward. The lesson from this case is to always have a back-up plan. Many situations like this will arise and I am glad to have learnt how to manage it. My back-up if the stent did not pass, was to ask interventional radiology to insert a nephrostomy. As the procedure was done in the morning, if it failed, there was an interventional radiology list that afternoon.

6.4   Always Maintain Patient Safety

It is important to remember, theatre time is precious but patient safety always comes first. One day I was taken from a theatre list in one hospital and asked to go and support the registrar on call, as the FY1 had to go to teaching and the FY2 was off sick. It is important that patient care and safety in these situations are maintained. It is also good if you can look for alternative solutions to problems where possible.

Know who to contact when you are in trouble, and if they are not helpful, contact someone who is. On one occasion, I had the most difficult stent I had ever encountered. Thankfully, I was on call with a supportive consultant. Prior to calling him, I had tried to pass a sensor, terumo and rio wire past a large impacted distal ureteric stone. With one phone call, he came in. As he walked into theatre, I had got the ureteroscope up the ureter and then managed to past the guidewire to the renal pelvis. It was still the most difficult stent I had ever encountered, but it was a supportive consultant that made the difference. A little bit of support goes a long way.

6.5   Reactions to Negative External Factors

Very often, what impacts any member of the team are their reactions to negative external factors. It is important to adopt a calm and controlled response mechanism. It is important for any team member to realise they are the sole custodian of my reaction to any given situation. It is important to let go off specific negative situations and focus on what can be learnt from them. Through mindfulness and a calm, balanced approach, it is important in these situations to let the negativity wash over you without leaving a mark. Develop a heightened ability to stand back and refocus on what is in front of you. Fighting against the reality of a given situation only leads to frustration and conflict. Letting go of any negativity in the workplace will lead to a more mature, calmer, at peace self. Furthermore, by becoming goal-orientated and outcome based in thinking, you can become more focused on the tasks at hand.

6.6   Work Closely with Your Team

Working closely with the consultant body and having a group of people who are supportive makes a huge difference. In many contexts it is possible to operate with peers at a "know" or "like" (from the know-like-trust-transact interaction continuum). True connection and therefore value comes from the higher level of "trust" and "transact". At any level in medicine, especially if more senior, you must be able to operate at the "transact" level. An environment with a high level of support and encouragement greatly improves morale and performance.

6.7   Always Be Accessible

Accessibility is a key part of Good Medical Practice. All medical staff need to be accessible to all team members. On one occasion, throughout the day the PA called me about several cases and results. The overall outcome was three nephrostomies placed in 1 day. At the end of the day—the interventional radiology unit was contacted to ensure all nephrostomies had gone in and that all the patients were stable. Following review of all the patients, all the nephrostomies were in and draining satisfactorily. It is important that any member of the team can approach you so that patient care and safety is maintained. Very often, when doctors are 'HALT-ed' meaning, hungry, angry, late, and tired, this can often result in adverse outcomes. It is important for doctors to be self-aware to prevent this from occurring.

6.8   Dealing with Conflict

Medicine can often present a harsh environment, but it is often the case of knowing how to deal with it. As a junior registrar, when on call with a particular consultant, I was told to 'just get on with the operation.' At the end of the operation, I didn't get any credit for successfully inserting the stents. Instead, I was told 'yes you can do that,' in a very abrupt manner. Despite this, always maintain good working professional relationships. My first interaction with this consultant at the start of the day, was light-hearted and jokey. It made this interaction so much easier. It is important when situations like this occur, to reflect on it with a clinical supervisor or educational supervisor. Trust is built on sincerity, consistency, competence, reliability, commitment, and integrity. A lack of acknowledgement of any of these factors in trust can damage the foundation for a good relationship. That is why it is so important to have a supportive clinical team.

6.9 Why We Need to Have Good Communication Between All Team Members

Patient safety is paramount and to maintain this you need a well-functioning team. When on call, I once had a critical unwell patient. This patient was so unwell, that they required input from four nursing staff and HCAs, myself, and my junior staff to just keep them stable. It was a case which required multidisciplinary multi-speciality input. The consultant was also called to review the patient. Given the strength of the relationship between the nursing staff and myself, we were able to save that patient. Anything I asked for was dealt with swiftly and promptly. At the end of the day, I wrote my thanks to the nursing sister on the ward as I couldn't have saved this patient alone. I also thanked the juniors very much for their input. They came running to help, even though they did not have to. It was due to the nature and strength of this relationship that the whole team came together, and the patient's life was saved. This emphasises how important it is to maintain good relationships with everyone.

6.10 Managing Juniors in Difficulty

As part of my training, I have conducted a self-assessment of emotional intelligence. It is important to be supportive of any team member who has family within another country. The ones that come into the category, that you need to keep an eye on, are those very often with family in another country. It was Goleman that first proposed the theory of emotional intelligence—self-awareness, self-management, social awareness, and relationship management. My juniors get treated like my children—I have an open-door policy so they can come and talk to me at any time. I was a little surprised one day, when one of my juniors looked very sad and came out with the fact that he had lost a cousin to suicide. He was in shock. To compound matters further, he was the man of his family here in England and also had a new baby to look after. The first step I took was letting the consultant body be aware of what had happened. The second was keeping an eye on him and letting him know that if he wanted to talk further, I was available. Over the next few weeks, he went through the steps of the grief reaction—the hardest part was having to deal with grief at the same time as looking after family and working a full-time clinical job. It was important to make sure he was getting enough rest, eating properly, and sleeping properly, which can be especially difficult when having to also care for a baby. Emotional intelligence is the most important lesson learnt here.

Communication Within a Theatre Team

7

Ruth Warne

7.1   Rationale for Effective Communication

Communication and human factors are elements of medical practice which are often, wrongly, overlooked. Poor communication can put patient safety at risk and create a poor working environment.

In 2009, the World Health Organization (WHO) introduced its guidelines for safe surgery. WHO estimated that over half of patient complications were arising from 'non-surgical', preventative causes. In its guideline, it introduced the 'WHO checklist' (Fig. 7.2), which allows the theatre team to share knowledge pre, intra and post-operatively. It aims to reduce preventable risk of harm to any patient entering the operating theatre environment.

Prior to its introduction, post-operative morbidity and mortality was 11.0% and 1.5% respectively.

Post introduction, these figures declined to 7.0% and 0.8% [1].

The checklist, or variations of, is now an integral part of theatre practice and one with which all clinicians and nurses should be familiar.

7.2   Elective Theatres

Every elective list requires discussion prior to its commencement. That is, the team in its entirety should discuss each case and decide on list order, prioritising patients according to clinical need.

The brief is an important meeting which provides the opportunity for the surgeon and anesthetist to state equipment and medication requirements (e.g., antibiotics,

R. Warne (✉)
Anaesthetics, East of England Deanery, Cambridge, UK

anticoagulation) and to voice any specific concerns that they may have concerning the anaesthetic or surgery.

7.3 Confidential Enquiries into Perioperative Deaths (CEPOD) Theatre ('*Emergencies*')

Every hospital has an operating theatre which is staffed 24 h a day to facilitate emergency 'life or limb saving' surgery. This theatre is available to all surgical specialties.

It is advisable to check local protocols on starting in a new hospital as to how this is locally managed. One theatre team and one anaesthetist is usually allocated to this theatre and all cases requiring urgent intervention MUST be discussed with the wider team involved.

7.4 Pre-operative Communication

CEPOD lists are at risk of being chaotic as they are at risk of constant change, depending on the severity of injury or clinical status of a patient. As such, it is helpful to provide as much detail as possible to the theatre team, and importantly, the CEPOD anesthetist, when informing them of the patient. *It is preferable to do this in person if possible.*

'SBAR' is a tried and tested method of communication and one with which most healthcare staff are familiar (Table 7.1).

In discussing the patient with the CEPOD anesthetist, it is useful to consider the following:

A patient's medical background provides crucial details about how well they will tolerate surgery and an anesthetic. Anesthetists are especially interested in any medical conditions which can compromise the airway or hemodynamics of a patient. As such, a detailed history of respiratory and cardiovascular disease is always helpful. From the medical history, the anesthetist will assign an 'American Association of Anesthesiologists' (ASA) grade, details of which are outlined in Fig. 7.1 [2]. This grade helps categories the severity of co-morbidities a patient has, which helps to assess their overall risk for an anesthetic and surgery.

Additional useful considerations to include in medical background:

Table 7.1 SBAR communication

S	Situation	Current situation of a patient Why does the patient need surgery? Why does the patient need surgery *now*? *Remember the mantra of 'life or limb saving' to help guide your communication.*
B	Background	Past medical history
A	Assessment	Communicate blood or imaging results which support
R	Recommendation	Operation which is to be performed Urgency of desired treatment

ASA PS Classification	Definition	Adult Examples, Including, but not Limited to:	Pediatric Examples, Including but not Limited to:
ASA I	A normal healthy patient	Healthy, non-smoking, no or minimal alcohol use	Healthy (no acute or chronic disease), normal BMI percentile for age
ASA II	A patient with mild systemic disease	Mild diseases only without substantive functional limitations. Current smoker, social alcohol drinker, pregnancy, obesity (30<BMI<40), well-controlled DM/HTN, mild lung disease	Asymptomatic congenital cardiac disease, well controlled dysrhythmias, asthma without exacerbation, well controlled epilepsy, non-insulin dependent diabetes mellitus, abnormal BMI percentile for age, mild/moderate OSA, oncologic state in remission, autism with mild limitations
ASA III	A patient with severe systemic disease	Substantive functional limitations: One or more moderate to severe diseases. Poorly controlled DM or HTN, COPD, morbid obesity (BMI ≥40), active hepatitis alcohol dependence or abuse, implanted pacemaker, moderate reduction of ejection fraction, ESRD undergoing regularly scheduled dialysis, history (>3 months) of MI, CVA, TIA, or CAD/stents.	Uncorrected stable congenital cardiac abnormality, asthma with exacerbation, poorly controlled epilepsy, insulin dependent diabetes mellitus, morbid obesity, malnutrition, severe OSA, oncologic state, renal failure, muscular dystrophy, cystic fibrosis, history of organ transplantation, brain/spinal cord malformation, symptomatic hydrocephalus, premature infant PCA <60 weeks, autism with severe limitations, metabolic disease, difficult airway, long term parenteral nutrition. Full term infants <6 weeks of age.
ASA IV	A patient with severe systemic disease that is a constant threat to life.	Recent (<3 months) MI, CVA, TIA or CAD/stents, ongoing cardiac ischemia or severe valve dysfunction, severe reduction of ejection fraction, shock, sepsis, DIC, ARD or ESRD not undergoing regularly scheduled dialysis	Symptomatic congenital cardiac abnormality, congestive heart failure, active sequelae of prematurity, acute hypoxic-ischemic encephalopathy, shock, sepsis, disseminated intravascular coagulation, automatic implantable cardioverter-defibrillator, ventilator dependence, endocrinopathy, severe trauma, severe respiratory distress, advanced oncologic state.
ASA V	A moribund patient who is not expected to survive without the operation	Ruptured abdominal/thoracic aneurysm, massive trauma, intracranial bleed with mass effect, ischemic bowel in the face of significant cardiac pathology or multiple organ/system dysfunction	Massive trauma, intracranial hemorrhage with mass effect, patient requiring ECMO, respiratory failure or arrest, malignant hypertension, decompensated congestive heart failure, hepatic encephalopathy, ischemic bowel or multiple organ/system dysfunction.
ASA VI	A declared brain-dead patient whose organs are being removed for donor purposes		

Fig. 7.1 American Association of Anaesthesiologists Anaesthetic classification scheme

7.5 Anti-coagulation

In some high-risk patients, general anaesthetic poses its challenges. As an example, in a patient with significant respiratory problems, there is a risk that the patient will be unable to breathe for themselves on waking. As an alternative, anesthetists frequently opt for 'regional blockade', that is, spinal anesthesia. One contraindication for this procedure is current anticoagulation.

7.6 'Nil by Mouth'

Aspiration during general anesthesia remains the highest cause of airway-related mortality [3]. The risk increases in emergency surgical patients. As such, it is useful to find out when a patient last ate or drank; this is to avoid undue risk of aspiration of stomach contents. Guideline's state >6 h for solids (including milk) and >2 h for clear fluids. If a patient is critically unwell and requires immediate surgery, anesthetists can perform a rapid sequence induction intubation which involves endotracheal intubation (over a slightly less invasive 'supraglottic' device) in the hope of reducing risk of aspiration. If a surgery can wait, it is preferable to do so to reduce the risk of aspiration.

7.7 Assessment

Providing information about a patient's current vital signs National Early Warning Score (NEWS) gives a good idea about the clinical urgency for surgical intervention. Blood samples and/or imaging results can further support this clinical picture.

7.8 Recommendation

The theatre team will need to know what procedure and equipment the surgeon will require. The anesthetist may be required to give prophylactic antibiotics prior to incision.

7.9 Peri and Intra-operative Communication

As previously mentioned, the 'WHO checklist' (Fig. 7.2) must be performed at the start of every operation. It is good practice to preface this check with a team introduction, which should follow the format: 'Name, Role, Grade'. All other communication must stop during this check.

It is crucial that anesthetist and surgeon communication continues throughout the time the patient is in theatre.

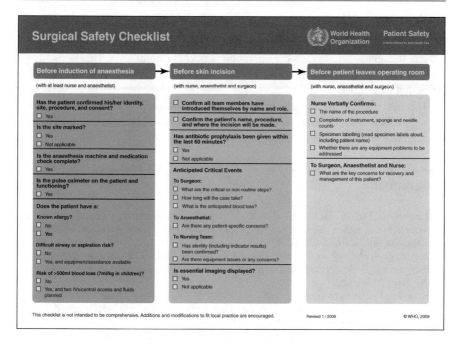

Fig. 7.2   Surgical Safety Checklist, World Health Organisation, 2009 [4]

7.10   "STARTING"

It is helpful for the operating surgeon to announce when they are commencing surgery. The anaesthetist can then confirm that the patient is suitably anaesthetised to tolerate surgical incision. This is a time when a patient may experience laryngospasm if they are not suitably anaesthetised or analgesed. This can cause airway obstruction. By confirming that surgery is starting, the anesthetist can administer more analgesia and be on 'high alert' for any compromise to the patient's airway.

7.11   "STOP"

If the anaesthetist asks the surgeon to stop surgery, it is vital this is done immediately.

Whilst most deviations in physiology can be managed without interruption to the surgeon, there are several situations which can arise which require immediate withdrawal of surgical stimulus in order to re-establish a safe physiological state. Should the anaesthetist ask for the surgeon to stop, it is important to withdraw surgical stimulus and only recommence once the anaesthetist has confirmed that it is safe to do so.

7.12 "Closing"

Inform the anaesthetist when the operation is near to completion. This allows them time to administer any final medication and to start preparing to wake the patient in a timely fashion.

The anaesthetist and surgeon have a unique relationship in medicine and should be a symbiotic one. By establishing good communication early in the relationship, it will make work both more effective and enjoyable.

References

1. Haynes AB, Weiser TG, Berry WR, et al. A surgical safety checklist to reduce morbidity and mortality in a global population. N Engl J Med. 2009;360:491–9. Accessed 14 Apr 2021. https://doi.org/10.1056/NEJMsa0810119.
2. American Society of Anesthesiologists ASA Physical Status Classification System. 2020. https://www.asahq.org/standards-and-guidelines/asa-physical-status-classification-system. Accessed 20 May 2021.
3. Robinson R, Davidson A. Aspiration under anesthesia: risk assessment and decision-making. Br J Anesth Continuing Educ Anesth Crit Care Pain. 2014;14(4):171–5. Accessed 29 May 2021. https://doi.org/10.1093/bjaceaccp/mkt053.
4. World Health Organization. Surgical Safety Checklist. 2009. http://apps.who.int/iris/bitstream/handle/10665/44186/9789241598590_eng_Checklist.pdf?sequence=2. Accessed 14 Apr 2021.

Digital Communications in Urology During the COVID-19 Pandemic

8

Karen Ventii, Sanchia S. Goonewardene, David Albala, and Aria Olumi

8.1 Introduction

Digital technology is an essential form of communication and information dissemination in healthcare. Traditionally, the healthcare industry has been slow to adopt digital communication. However, that reluctance is rapidly fading, particularly in the post-COVID-19 era, as healthcare systems and the entire industry have made the digital transformation. The rationale for participating in digital communication comes from a need to expand patient's access to information and do so with greater transparency. It is important for healthcare professionals to have a working knowledge of available digital communication options and how they can be utilized in clinical practice. For example, platforms like Twitter provide opportunities for physicians to interact, collaborate, and exchange information with colleagues. We aimed to assess perceptions and attitudes towards digital communication amongst urologists. In this review, we summarize our findings and provides guidance on how to avoid some of the problems that digital communication can bring.

K. Ventii (✉)
Harvard University, Boston, MA, USA
e-mail: karen@thegoldstargrp.com

S. S. Goonewardene
Department of Urology, The Princess Alexandra Hospital, Harlow, UK

D. Albala
Associated Medical Professionals, Syracuse, NY, USA
e-mail: dalbala@ampofny.com

A. Olumi
Beth Israel Deaconess Medical Center, Harvard Medical School, Boston, MA, USA
e-mail: aolumi@bidmc.harvard.edu

© The Author(s), under exclusive license to Springer Nature Switzerland AG 2022
F. Motiwala et al. (eds.), *When Things Go Wrong In Urology*,
https://doi.org/10.1007/978-3-031-13658-0_8

8.2   Methods

We designed an 18-question survey to assess usage and perceived usefulness of digital communication tools and distributed it online to urologists across the country. Two hundred and sixty-seven urologists participated in the survey from September 1–30, 2020.

8.3   Results

Participant ages were equally distributed amongst those in their 30s (18%), 40s (26.5%), 50s (23.5%), and 60s (20%). Eleven percent were in their 70s. Fifty-five percent were academic practitioners while 31% were from the community. Fellows and residents made up 3% and 2%, respectively and 68% of respondents had been in practice for at least 10 years.

The survey revealed that many respondents prefer to receive information online (41%) via their computer (52%)—mostly in the form of online PDFs (45%) or web articles (33%). Online videos were preferred by 7.5% of respondents. In person interactions were the next most popular way to receive medical information, either at a conference (31.5%) or from an in-person meeting (17%), while virtual conferences were preferred by 11% of respondents as a way to receive information. iPhones (79%) were the preferred device followed by Windows devices (11%) and Android devices (7.5%).

Social media sites like Twitter, Facebook, and Instagram were used by 34%, 26%, and 9% of participants respectively, whereas 24% did not use social media at all. One respondent preferred crowd sourcing information from medical expert groups on Facebook and other social media.

Forty-five percent preferred using email to communicate with other medical colleagues. An equal percentage preferred text and in person communication (19% each). Nine percent prefer phone while a smaller percentage preferred online messaging. When it came to patient communication, 63% preferred doing so in-person, followed by 13% over the phone and 10% via email.

COVID-19 had a huge impact on urologists' approach to communicating with medical colleagues and patients; in particular, it reduced in-person meetings and increased telemedicine/telehealth. During the pandemic, Zoom became a popular communication tool in use by 88% of respondents, followed by Webex (27%), Microsoft Teams (22%), GoTo Meeting (17%), and Skype (9%). Respondents also reported having more emails and gateway messages during the pandemic.

8.4   Discussion

This online survey of 267 urologists highlights how digital technology is changing the way health care professionals communicate with colleagues and patients.

The biggest challenge facing urologists with the use of digital technologies in media communications is the lack of universal guidance/oversight on use of digital technologies (59%); in particular, the security concerns on digital devices (e.g., through passwords or encryption). Maintaining privacy of information came in second, with 31% of the votes. Other challenges with increased digital communications are that images cannot be communicated as well, some patients are unable to adapt to new technologies, there are more barriers for non-English speaking patients, and in some cases more off-hours work for physicians.

However, the increase in use of digital technology has not been entirely negative. Some respondents felt that it has increased efficiency of communication and forced telemedicine meetings to become more structured (e.g., clarifying the goal of the discussion, having fewer open-ended discussion) and resulted in some urologists having more time on their hands (given the stay-at-home orders) during the height of the pandemic.

The survey results reinforced the impact of the COVID-19 pandemic on reducing in-person contact and causing urologists to have more willingness to communicate online, which some believed was far better for initial visits and follow-ups (while understanding the need for in-person visit at some point in the middle).

Specifically, the disruption triggered by COVID-19 has 'virtualised' many aspects of the patient–physician engagement lifecycle. The initial patient screening and scheduling process, which was traditionally done via phone call, is now increasingly done via web, app, or chatbot, given the risks posed by in-person engagement between patients infected by COVID-19 and caregivers without adequate N-95 masks, gloves, or PPE for protection. Likewise, the patient history and data capture step, is also increasingly done via online forms, apps or chatbots. The initial patient–physician appointment remains more valuable when done in-person however, follow-up appointments are now done via telehealth unless in-person is imperative.

When used wisely and prudently, digital technology offers the potential to promote effective communication amongst urologists and with their patients. However, there are some pitfalls, particularly if these technologies are used carelessly. Clear guidelines issued by health care organizations and professional societies are warranted to provide sound and useful principles to help avoid pitfalls.

Legal Records and Documentation

9

Faiz Motiwala, Hanif Motiwala,
and Sanchia S. Goonewardene

Clinical records may be held electronically, manually or both. Good record-keeping is paramount to delivering high-quality care, particularly with the involvement of multiple clinicians and teams.

Medical records provide:

- Patient support and continuity of care
- Documentation to support clinical audit or research
- Capability to meet legal requirements
- Necessary facts in cases of complaints or clinical negligence claims

These records include a variety of documents such as letters, clinical notes (handwritten or typed), emails, lab results, photographs, video/audio recordings, printouts from medical equipment and consent forms. As they contain identifiable information, all records are confidential and are subject to the Data Protection Act.

Significant areas of documentation include:

- Clinic appointments/letters
- Multi-disciplinary team meetings
- Investigation results
- Ward round entries

F. Motiwala
Queen Elizabeth Hospital, Woolwich, UK
e-mail: faiz.motiwala@nhs.net

H. Motiwala
Department of Urology, Southend University Hospital, Southend, UK

S. S. Goonewardene (✉)
Department of Urology, The Princess Alexandra Hospital, Harlow, UK

© The Author(s), under exclusive license to Springer Nature
Switzerland AG 2022
F. Motiwala et al. (eds.), *When Things Go Wrong In Urology*,
https://doi.org/10.1007/978-3-031-13658-0_9

- Review of a deteriorating patient
- Consent forms
- Operation notes

Despite the importance of documentation, it remains a low priority for some health-care professionals. Notes may be poorly maintained, not readily available, or simply not even used. Sometimes there may be inconsistencies, illegible writing and surprisingly offensive language/slang. Poor record keeping is a major factor of litigation cases [1].

The GMC advise for all documentation to be clear, accurate and legible, with the record made at made at the time the events happen or as soon as possible following the event [2]. The record should also include relevant clinical findings, decisions made and agreed action (with the responsible clinician named), information provided to the patients, any medications prescribed, investigations or treatment planned, and who is making the record in addition to when. The record should be an accurate reflection of the events that have transpired (Fig. 9.1).

While an obvious point, a surprising number of medical notes are illegible. This makes it particularly difficult should the notes be required for defence in a claim or if you may need to recall an event that occurred years ago. Even worse is that if other cannot read your writing they may find difficulty in interpreting your assessment or plan for the patient compromising good continuity of care. Abbreviations can further complicate the picture; RTA—road traffic accident or renal tubular acidosis? PID—pelvic inflammatory disease or prolapsed intervertebral disc? These may be obvious to you or make sense in the context of your experience, but this is not always the case for others reading the entry; it is ultimately clearer and safer to avoid abbreviations with multiple meanings in medical record entries [3].

A grave issue arises from altering documentation for the purpose of hiding deficiencies; these are practically impossible to defend. If there is a new finding or you realise you wrote something incorrectly, these should be scored out with a single line (such that the original text is legible), with the correct portion following it. The incorrect portion should be marked as being incorrect, or with the note 'wrong patient' if it was written in the wrong notes and the correct portion marked with the

---

- Be legible, clear and complete
- Avoid ambiguous abbreviations
- Avoid altering an entry or disguising an addition
- Avoid unnecessary comments
- Keep language used simple
- Check dictated letters and notes
- Check reports

Fig. 9.1 Tips for good record keeping

updated date, time and signature. Furiously scrubbing out words to be ineligible only adds suspicion.

Some clinicians opt to dictate their ward round entries for their secretary to type up and place into the relevant patient notes. In these circumstances it is the responsibility of the clinician to ensure the typed information is correct and sign them appropriately. This is particularly useful for long-term records. A disadvantage to this method may be the time elapsed prior to the entry being placed in the patient's notes. This can be several days. The ward round team may be aware of the plan, but it may not be clear to the nursing staff if there is poor handover, or the on-call doctor if they are asked to see the patient. A contemporaneous handwritten record would be beneficial for this situation, but ultimately does duplicates the amount of work.

Some trusts use electronic systems with typed notes or provide the option for this. While this comes with the advantage of legibility, these may suffer from their own problems such as slow or inefficient systems and the time required to find a computer and upload these entries.

Should a complaint or clinical negligence claim arise, the defence will rely highly on these documents. A lack of information or failure to read the relevant clinical notes can result in serious consequences to the livelihood of the patient and increases the probability of complaints or litigation. There should be comprehensive information to allow for the continuation of care by a different clinician. Should essential information be missing or unclear, cases may be lost which might have been won. For all intents and purposes, if the event is not documented, then it has not occurred.

9.1 Operation Notes

Operation notes are subject to the same requirements and recommendations as all other records. The responsibility of the operation notes lies with the operating surgeon—these should be clear, comprehensive and include unexpected problems/complications. It is common practice to leave the junior to write it which may be useful for their education or learning, or it may be done out of courtesy and to save the senior/consultant time (especially if the junior is trusted to do so). It is however the responsibility of the consultant/senior-most surgeon to ensure the note is accurate and detailed.

A picture is worth a thousand words and diagrams can be extremely helpful. Phrases such as 'straightforward...' or 'standard prostatectomy' are inadequate to surmise the entire operation. Operations have been described as such and have resulted in complications, with a lack of defence in subsequent litigation resulting in successful negligence claims. Technique used and layers should be identified as well as method of closure. Drains or catheters should be clearly mentioned or included in the diagram to guide the post-operative care period. The post-operative plan should be clear for even the junior-most surgical team member to act upon. This should include the plan for drains/catheters, antibiotics, DVT prophylaxis, anticoagulation and potential discharge plan if appropriate (Fig. 9.2).

- Clear (preferably typed) operative notes for each procedure
- The notes should include:
    - Date and time
    - Elective/emergency
    - Names of operating surgeons and assistant
    - Name of theatre anaesthetist
    - Operative procedure
    - Incision
    - Operative diagnosis
    - Operative findings
    - Problems/complications (if applicable)
    - Extra procedures performed and why if so
    - Details of tissue removed, added, or altered
    - Details of prosthesis used, including the serial numbers of prostheses and other implanted materials
    - Details of closure technique
    - Anticipated blood loss
    - Antibiotic prophylaxis (where applicable)
    - DVT prophylaxis (where applicable)
    - Detailed postoperative care instructions
    - Signature

Fig. 9.2 The Royal College of Surgeons England recommendations for operation notes [4]

9.2 Delayed Presentations and the Importance of Documentation

We have experienced a case of testicular torsion in which the patient claimed that from arrival to hospital and subsequent surgical exploration was the cause for his testicle to become necrotic and necessitate orchidectomy. On review of the records and documentation, the patient had presented to the Emergency Department after 10 h of pain. The time from the patient's arrival to review by a urology registrar was 20 min, with the time to scrotal exploration 60 min from the patient's presentation to the Emergency Department. The prompt review and clear documentation by the urology registrar of the patient's timeline and the timing of their review, with additional proof from operating theatre timings, allowed for simple defence of the case. This was arguably in fact a very good time from presentation to surgical exploration.

References

1. Goodwin H. Litigation and surgical practice in the UK. Br J Surg. 2000;87(8):977–9.
2. General Medical Council. The duties of a doctor registered with the General Medical Council. 2013. www.gmc-uk.org/guidance/good_medical_practice/duties_of_a_doctor.asp. Accessed Mar 2020.
3. Mathioudakis A, Rousalova I, Gagnat AA, Saad N, Hardavella G. How to keep good clinical records. Breathe (Sheffield, England). 2016;12(4):369–73.
4. Royal College of Surgeons. 1.3 Record your work clearly, accurately and legibly—Royal College of Surgeons. https://www.rcseng.ac.uk/standards-and-research/gsp/domain-1/1-3-record-your-work-clearly-accurately-and-legibly/. Accessed Apr 2020.

Consent

Faiz Motiwala, Hanif Motiwala,
and Sanchia S. Goonewardene

Every individual maintains the right to their bodily integrity. Consent allows the breach of this integrity for the purpose of providing adequate healthcare. It forms the basis of our daily practice. It forms part of the duty of care to inform patients of the options for treatment, outcomes, complications and alternatives. A failure to consent a patient is a breach of that duty of care.

Consent can be either [1]:

- Implied e.g. a patient visiting and vocalising their medical problem, or undressing themselves for an exam.
- Expressed e.g. orally or written.

In principle, it is not the written document that serves as value, but rather the exchange of information that occurs during the process of consent. Whilst both forms of consent are equally valid, a written document serves as evidence.

Consent is a leading cause of medico-legal cases filed. It relates to patients frequently arguing their lack of knowledge or being misled surrounding the risks of the procedure; that they would not have undergone it had they understood it. Much of consent thus relates to good communication between the clinician and the patient [2, 3].

F. Motiwala
Queen Elizabeth Hospital, Woolwich, UK
e-mail: faiz.motiwala@nhs.net

H. Motiwala
Department of Urology, Southend University Hospital, Southend, UK

S. S. Goonewardene (✉)
Department of Urology, The Princess Alexandra Hospital, Harlow, UK

F. Motiwala et al. (eds.), *When Things Go Wrong In Urology*,
https://doi.org/10.1007/978-3-031-13658-0_10

There are three components to a valid consent:

1. Capacity—the patient must legally be competent. The patient must comprehend the nature of the proposed action. Various factors influence these such as age, mental state, physical state, intellect, reason for performing the procedure, and an understanding of risks vs. benefits.
2. Voluntariness—the consent is given freely.
3. Appropriateness—that the procedure is not unduly and only that which is required is performed. It is only acceptable to perform additional acts or procedures such that it cannot be delayed e.g. life-saving procedures.

It can be difficult to predict the nature or capacity of some patients and this should be accounted for. Although assumed in everyone, a patient found to be lacking the capacity to comprehend or consent to that procedure should have the procedure performed in their best interest. A patient may lack the capacity in certain areas, but have it retained in others. This should be assessed for each individual scenario. Patients must also receive all relevant information relating to the procedure prior to proceeding.

Although rare there can be claims from patients who feel they were 'coerced' into the procedure, rendering the consent invalid. Such cases are rare, but patients can feel this to be the case, or have difficulty in saying no [4]. Others such as relatives or friends can considerably influence their decision. Patients must always be given the opportunity to refuse treatment and the right to a second opinion, regardless of one's concern for their best interest. As such, patients must always be offered the option of no treatment, with the risks and benefits of that option also fully explained [1, 5].

10.1 Consent Post-Montgomery

The process of consent has continuously evolved, and the Montgomery case in 2015 defined a new era of informed consent [6]. The risk of shoulder dystocia occurring during vaginal delivery was not discussed with Ms. Montgomery, who had Type 1 Diabetes Mellitus and was in her first pregnancy. The responsible consultant stated the risk of shoulder dystocia in a woman with diabetes mellitus was 10%, with the risk of consequent injury from said dystocia to be 0.2% for brachial plexus injury and less than 0.1% for hypoxic brain injury. Due to the low risk in her opinion, it was not discussed with the patient. The consultant did however highlight that the risk would have been mentioned if the specific question had been asked (referring to the ruling of Lord Diplock in Sidaway in that if a specific question was asked, it should be answered). However, doctors cannot expect patients to ask specific questions relating to these procedures as it requires a basic medical knowledge of the procedure itself, something we should not expect a non-medical professional to have.

There were failed appeals in the Court of Session and Inner Houses prior to the case being heard before the UK Supreme Court in July 2014. This case was presented before Seven Justices (which is in fact the number of justices required to change or overrule a previous House of Lords ruling i.e. the ruling in Sidaway). All seven justices supported the appeal and the ruling was overturned.

This new ruling also supported the concept of material risk proposed by Lord Scarman in juxtaposition to the Sidaway ruling. That is, material risk is that which is deemed to have significance by the individual patient as opposed to that deemed by the doctor.

To facilitate this extensive process, several surgeons have begun opting for consent clinics; clinics dedicated to consenting patients. These reduce time detracted from regular outpatient clinics and enables dedicated time for focused conversations relating to the procedure. The added benefit of these clinics is obtaining consent well in advance of the procedure. This provides the opportunity for the patient to consider their options, consider any questions and contact you if there are additional questions or concerns. It also allows the opportunity to ensure any pre-operative checks have been performed or will be performed. The consent can be facilitated with additional written information, leaflets, audio-visual/multi-media presentations and more [3]. The disadvantage of these is the extra clinic slots required and time detracted from other duties. Some departments may also not be large enough to warrant the need for consent clinics.

10.2 Case 1: Informed Consent—Chronic Scrotal Pain Post-vasectomy

A 39-year-old man requested a vasectomy and was reviewed by a urologist for the procedure to be performed in day case surgery under general anaesthetic. The patient signed a consent form which included a list of all the risks and complications. The operation note was legible and clear with a detailed explanation of the procedure. Post-operatively the patient experienced scrotal bruising and swelling but resolved within 2 weeks. Four months later the patient presented to his GP with chronic scrotal pain on one side and was prescribed oral analgesics. This pain failed to respond and the patient was referred by the GP to the pain team in hospital; higher doses of oral analgesia, local anaesthesia and steroids provided no benefit. The patient sued the urologist for clinical negligence claiming this complication was not discussed with him and the procedure was performed poorly. The claim failed due to clear evidence from the surgeon's diligent documentation and clear operation note proving due care and attention when he performed the operation.

10.2.1 Chaperones and Documentation

Vasectomy is one of the commonest causes for complaint to arise. Despite being a relatively short and simple procedure, every aspect of the consultation should be completed with diligence and documentation is vital. The presence of a chaperone is highly recommended and additional copies that can be given to the patient safeguard against issues arising from allegations of altering documentation such as that suggested by the patient in this case. By thorough documentation, the urologist proved that there was no breach of duty and thus medical negligence could not be claimed.

To avoid such situations arising it is imperative the patient understands the procedure that is due to be performed, with an understanding of the risks vs. the benefits and clear documentation of the conversation that has taken place. For this reason, the authors recommend the use of leaflets, particularly from the British Association of Urological Surgeons (BAUS) to support discussions and allow the patient to have a better understanding both of their procedure and the follow-up. The presence of a chaperone facilitates these discussions.

10.3 Case 2: Failure of Vasectomy

In a case published by the Medical Protection Society, a 35-year-old male consulted a urologist over the phone for vasectomy [7]. The urologist briefly explained the procedure over the phone including bleeding, infection and chronic scrotal pain. He then sent the patient the hospital admission and consent form to bring on the day of the operation. Upon admission to the ward, he met another urologist who introduced herself, checked his signature and consent form informing him that he would be able to go home later that day. On discharge he was only advised to get a sperm count organised by his GP in 12 weeks. He claimed there was no practical advice or counselling provided regarding contraception. The patient visited his GP who was surprised to hear of the operation. He requested a pathology lab test for sperm analysis and advised the patient to contact the urology department for the results. He had however failed to label the semen analysis as post-vasectomy. The patient attempted to contact the clinic but was unable to speak to any doctors. The secretary informed him that the report stated "normal"—the patient interpreted that this meant the operation was successful. Unfortunately, the patient's wife became pregnant and the significance of the semen analysis report became evident. The patient claimed against all doctors involved. It could not be defended and the case was settled for a moderate sum.

10.3.1 Communication and Pre-operative Counselling

Vasectomy is a safe and effective means of male sterilisation. Although a simple procedure, it has the potential for complications or failure and is one of the most common sources of litigation in urology. Medical negligence can be claimed if there was failure and inadequate counselling to the patient prior to the procedure. Reasons for vasectomy failure include:

1. Unprotected intercourse immediately following vasectomy
2. Late recanalisation
3. Technical failure

Patients should be counselled on the procedure, with an explanation of all potential risks/complications including failure. They should be informed that while it is the most effective form of male sterilisation, there is the chance they will remain fertile. They should also be informed what will be required of them post-procedure. A vasectomy is one of the few procedures where the simplicity of the procedure is not proportional to the detailed consent and counselling required.

The counselling should be done in an appropriate setting which allows the surgeon to explain the procedure in due detail and the patient able to ask questions. Telephone consults are convenient and useful for discussing simple cases. The caveat to these is the lack of rapport one might develop from an outpatient clinic review and the inability to examine or see the patient. While consenting patients is feasible through these means, this discussion must allow adequate exchange of information. Although not an element of the operation itself, this exchange of information should also include what is expected of the patient in the follow-up period and what they need to be mindful of. In the first case the complications and operation note were clearly documented which served as strong evidence in the claim. Within the second case it is unlikely the patient was provided all relevant information. Upon admission to the ward the second urologist performing the operation should have checked that the patient understood the operation as listed on the consent form and iterated what would be required post-operatively. Confirmation of consent is especially important in these cases when the initial consent was performed in a telephone consultation and the operating surgeon was not the one who initially consented. Had the risks of vasectomy including failure rate been re-iterated, either due to failure to remove adequate sections of both vasa or due to re-canalisation, it would have reduced the risk of the patient making a claim.

The following risks/complications should be highlighted [8, 9]

Early
- Wound infection
- Bruising and scrotal swelling
- Haematoma
- Haematospermia following first few ejaculations post-procedure
- Epididymo-orchitis
- Early recanalisation (~3–6 months post-vasectomy)

Late
- Chronic testicular pain
- Vas granulomas
- Late/delayed failure causing pregnancy

Typically, it takes approximately 3 months (or 20–25 ejaculates) post-procedure prior to sterility being achieved. This is the amount of time required for the live sperm to be eliminated from the epididymis. Patients should be informed of this and to avoid unprotected sexual intercourse in the first 3 months. This should also be clearly documented. Sterility should be confirmed by two post-operative semen samples with the absence of live sperm.

10.3.2 Bruising, Scrotal Swelling and Haematospermia

Although a minor and common consequence of the operation, your patient will be appreciative of being informed and are less likely to be alarmed when they note haematospermia, or some bruising and swelling in the scrotal area. On the contrary they may be pleased that it is not as bad as they thought it to be and will often be reassured by the explanation that the bruising typically resolves in 2 weeks. The occasional ones that do not (~1–2%) may progress to haematoma and require drainage, but this is an acceptable and a known complication of the operation provided they are aware of the risk.

10.3.3 Early Recanalisation

Recanalisation can occur either early or late. Early recanalisation or failure occurs within 3–6 months of the procedure. Sperm counts may initially decrease post-procedure but this levels off and may even increase. It is confirmed by post-operative semen analysis identifying motile sperm.

10.3.4 Late/Delayed Failure Causing Pregnancy

Late failure is defined as a pregnancy in the partner of a patient who has undergone vasectomy, where the two initial post-operative semen analyses were azoospermic, but the samples at the time of pregnancy confirm the presence of motile sperm. Despite the low incidence, it has drastic consequences.

The soft scar tissue at the end of the vas deferens may form tiny passages enabling sperm to travel through bypassing the obstruction. Techniques to reduce the risk of this include the use of either non-absorbable sutures or clips, interposing the cut end of the vas deferens away from each other (though this may increase complication rate of vasectomy), or cautery of the inside of the vas deferens.

10.3.5 Surgical Technique

Lastly, technical failure can also occur whereby the surgeon fails to identify the vas deferens correctly or fails to seal the vas deferens. This is more likely to occur in cases of aberrant anatomy or in patients who have had previous scrotal surgery that obscures usual anatomy. Patients with prior scrotal surgery should be informed of the increased risk of failure. This will result in persistent/normal sperm count in analyses post-procedure.

10.4   Case 3: A Nephrectomy Performed Without Consent

In another case published by the Medical Protection Society, a middle aged female with a background of cystinuria, consulted her urologist due to an episode of renal colic [10]. She had already underwent several open and laparoscopic procedures for stone removal from her left kidney and ureter and continued to form a new stone approximately every 8 weeks. An intravenous pyelogram demonstrated a large radiolucent stone in the left renal pelvis. She was advised that the stone would not be suitable for extracorporeal shockwave lithiotripsy (ESWL) as it was cysteine and lithotripters available locally were not capable for treating it. She was advised for nephrolithotomy instead. She underwent surgical exploration however the urologist found the kidney to be small and contracted. Following removal of the calculus he was unable to surgically reconstitute the kidney. The ureter had also been damaged during dissection, with the distal portion not amenable for surgical anastomosis. He made the decision to perform a nephrectomy. Subsequently the patient sued the surgeon for negligence. She argued that:

1. She had not given consent for nephrectomy.
2. She alleged the urology consultant never visited her post-operatively and that another member of staff had informed her that she had undergone nephrectomy.
3. She had not received an explanation from the consultant urologist as to why it was necessary.

The urologist claimed he had visited her in the immediate post-operative period but admitted she may not remember due to the effects of the general anaesthetic. In his opinion he felt that leaving the kidney in situ in such a situation could have led to complications such as urinary fistula, urinoma, abscess requiring further surgeries and worsening morbidity. He also stated that the post-operative care was taken over by his staff and he was easily contactable in case of any post-operative problems. The case could not be defended and was settled in court for the equivalent of £28,000 plus costs.

10.4.1 Communication and Selection of Management

There arose two issues from this case; the choice of management and communication to the patient. The role of nephrectomy in cystinuria is considered as a final step and in the presence of obstruction and infection. Alternative treatment modalities were not offered nor discussed with the patient. Understandably the decision was made based upon intra-operative findings, however the possibilities of medical management were not explored prior to the surgery and the procedure was not necessary at that particular time. Consequently, there was a lack of information provided to the patient with no warning regarding the possibility of nephrectomy.

It forms good practice to review your patient post-operatively. While not necessary in every case, the fact that he performed a procedure not previously discussed with the patient necessitates a clear formal explanation to the patient. Two of the points she had raised revolved around a lack of information from the surgeon and that fact that she did not recall him ever reviewing her. Had he visited her at more appropriate time, and taken the time to review, clearly explain to her what had transpired and the reasons for doing so, she may have been more accepting of the outcome.

This case also highlights the importance of the three aspects of consent; capacity, information and voluntariness. The latter two aspects were not fulfilled as the patient was not provided adequate information and consequently, she did not agree to the nephrectomy that was performed. Had the options been discussed with the patient and a treatment modality agreed following such discussion, the patient would ultimately not have made a claim and most importantly, she would have received ideal treatment.

10.5 Case 4: Failure to Inform About Outcomes and Alternative Treatments for Treatment of Bladder Outflow Obstruction

A 60-year-old man presented to the urology outpatient clinic with symptoms of hesitancy, poor urinary flow, increased frequency and nocturia. He found the symptoms of nocturia to be particularly bothersome to his quality-of-life. These symptoms had been present for over a year. Urinary flow rates or post-void residuals were not performed. Imaging of the upper urinary tract was not performed. A flexible cystoscopy was arranged in which the urologist noted an enlarged prostate and the patient was subsequently booked for a transurethral resection of the prostate under general anaesthesia. The procedure was explained to the patient though there was no documentation of complications or outcomes following the procedure.

He went on to have this operation under the care of a different surgeon who performed a hasty review of the patient and consent procedure as he was running late for the list. Intra-operatively he noted that the bladder neck was very high, though the prostate was only mildly enlarged. The surgeon performed the procedure, and the post-operative stay was uncomplicated. The patient did notice a subjective improvement in his urinary flow however he had ongoing persisting symptoms of nocturia and urinary frequency. He also unfortunately developed retrograde ejaculation for which he had not been warned about, nor was this documented in the consent form. He was reviewed again in clinic for his persisting symptoms almost a year after his initial operation. The patient then went on to have urinary flow studies and the pattern was suggestive of a urethral stricture. He went on to have another rigid cystoscopy in which a bladder neck stricture was identified and treated. Despite an improvement in urinary flow, he continued to have urinary symptoms and retrograde ejaculation. The patient sued complaining that he not been warned of failure of treatment or development of retrograde ejaculation, and no alternative options i.e., drug therapy was offered to him. The patient was successful in his claim.

10.5.1 Inadequate Investigation, Discussion of Treatment Options and Consent

This case highlights a lack of appropriate and complete investigation for the patient's symptoms. Beyond the urological problems for why one may experience these symptoms, the urologist had not even explored or documented potential medical causes for the patient's symptoms. While not necessarily relevant to this case, there are many referrals in practice where there has been inadequate work-up of the patient prior to specialist referral. Causes such as poorly controlled diabetes, congestive heart failure, medications and even excessive fluid intake prior to sleep can be culprits for patients' symptoms of urinary frequency and nocturia!

Beyond this, there was no initial assessment of urinary flow rate therefore it is impossible to know whether there was objectively a reduced flow rate or inadequate bladder emptying. Measurement of urinary flow is simple and allows for objective measurement of improvement following surgical intervention. The surgeon should have also asked the patient to complete the 'International prostate symptom score' (IPSS) when aware of the prostatic enlargement. There were other elements which were not performed such as a recorded digital rectal examination, either in the initial documentation or alongside the findings of the flexible cystoscopy. These are all recommended in the European Association of Urology (EAU) Guidelines in the management of non-neurogenic male LUTS [11].

Without any imaging there was no proper assessment of the upper urinary tract or evaluation of prostate size. Although not likely, there may have been other findings such as bladder stones or consequences of long-standing chronic bladder outlet obstruction such as hydronephrosis or ureteric dilatation. An ultrasound scan is a simple non-invasive means of obtaining some basic information about the anatomy of urinary tract that can be in support of any provisional diagnosis or treatment plan, particularly prior to proceeding with surgical treatment.

Alternative treatment options were not discussed with the patient. These options included the initial watchful waiting or medical treatment such as an alpha blocker and 5-alpha reductase inhibitor, permanent catheterisation (albeit this is certainly not ideal for this case) or alternative surgical treatments e.g., holmium laser enucleation therapy (HoLEP). Discussions of all alternative treatment options, outcomes and risks can seem a hassle particularly in a busy outpatient clinic, and sometimes the last thing you may feel like doing might be to drag on the consultation, and instead get a patient out of clinic as fast as possible. However, patients rely on your recommendations to make the best decision and that decision however well your intentions, should be one made by the patient after their consideration of all options. It relies on you investing the time to discuss *all* potential alternatives, outcomes and risks.

It is also essential to be as comprehensive as possible in discussions with patients regarding complications or risks. Not listing retrograde ejaculation (or sexual dysfunction for the matter) on the consent form for a TURP was a significant omission on the surgeon's part, whether it was due to forgetfulness or because of the rushed process as he was running late. The consent process should never be rushed. In some situations, it is also important to paint a realistic picture for the patient that an operation may not improve *all* of their symptoms and that there are real risks of proceeding with any operation, however minor these risks or however many hundreds of operations you may perform every year.

Lastly, the follow-up period of 1 year for post-void residual bladder scans and flow rate studies is too long and would have only contributed to the patient's misgivings about the operation. A follow-up period of 3–6 months would have been more appropriate.

10.6   A Word on Circumcision and 'Minor Operations'

Circumcision is a common source of complaints within urology. A general recurring theme of complaints from adult circumcision relate to cosmetic outcome or its effects on sexual function. Problems can arise due to the disparity between what the surgeon or patient deem to be an acceptable outcome. In addition to the BAUS procedure specific forms, this is one procedure in which providing additional detail to the patients can greatly reduce this disparity between surgeon and patient.

As highlighted earlier, it is important to provide a realistic idea of what to expect following an operation, or in this case circumcision. Patients often believe their organ will look perfect even as they are sat in the recovery room just waking up from the procedure! Warn them that this is not the case. The immediate post-operative period can be uncomfortable with some pain or discomfort. They might note significant bruising or swelling around the penis which takes time to settle. Warning them in advance makes it much easier to reassure a patient of a normal post-operative event as opposed to an unwelcome complication.

The final cosmetic appearance of the penis is not always a good outcome. This can especially be so for cases where the underlying pathology is balanitis xerotica obliterans. The marked fibrous reactions can make the surgery much more technically difficult and lead to a poorer cosmetic result regardless of how good the surgical technique. A change in sensation of the penis is also common. Loss of or heightened sensitivity can lead to increased or reduced enjoyment from sex, depending on the patient's circumstances.

The procedure is a reminder that consent for minor procedures should be equally as detailed as consent for complex or major operations. For a major operation, patients and their relatives are often more accepting of the complications, especially if the patient was sick to begin with. Conversely for smaller procedures, patients (and surgeons who have been lulled into a false sense of security) do not entertain the possibilities of complications after minor surgery. Going through the outcomes, putting it into perspective for the patient and *documenting all of this* significantly improves your standard of care.

10.7   Summary

- Consent is a process/discussion. A written document is merely evidence that the discussion has taken place.
- Consent requires the presence of capacity, voluntariness, and appropriateness.

- The consent should be taken within the context of the patient's individual background, knowledge, culture and interest.
- Leaflets should be used, such as from the BAUS website to support discussions of consent.
- A chaperone should be used where possible, particularly for intimate examinations.
- Alternative options including no intervention should be offered with the discussion clearly documented.
- Patients should be provided with realistic expectations following their surgery.
- Additional copies of consent should be given to the patient.
- Patients should be provided details to contact their surgeon via their secretary or acceptable alternative for complications relating to the procedure.
- Use of dedicated consent clinics should be considered in departments of appropriate sizes.

References

1. Satyanarayana Rao KH. Informed consent: an ethical obligation or legal compulsion? J Cutan Aesthet Surg. 2008;1(1):33–5.
2. Hall DE, Prochazka AV, Fink AS. Informed consent for clinical treatment. CMAJ. 2012;184(5):533–40.
3. Schenker Y, Fernandez A, Sudore R, et al. Interventions to improve patient comprehension in informed consent for medical and surgical procedures: a systematic review. Med Decis Making. 2011;31:151–73.
4. Lavelle-Jones C, Byrne DJ, Rice P, et al. Factors affecting quality of informed consent. BMJ. 1993;306:885–90.
5. Hutson MM, Blaha JD. Patients' recall of preoperative instruction for informed consent for an operation. J Bone Joint Surg Am. 1991;73(2):160–2.
6. Montgomery v Lanarkshire Health Board [2015] SC 11 [2015] 1 AC 1430.
7. Medical Protection Society: When normal is wrong. 2016. https://www.medicalprotection.org/malaysia/casebook-resources/case-reports/case-reports/row-when-normal-is-wrong. Accessed Jun 2020.
8. Awsare NS, Krishnan J, Boustead GB, Hanbury DC, McNicholas TA. Complications of vasectomy. Ann R Coll Surg Engl. 2005;87(6):406–10.
9. Sharlip ID, Belker AM, Honig S, et al. Vasectomy: AUA guideline. J Urol. 2012;188:2482.
10. Medical Protection Society: Consent not given for nephrectomy. 2006. https://www.medical-protection.org/uk/articles/consent-not-given-for-nephrectomy. Accessed Jun 2020.
11. European Association of Urology: Management of non-neurogenic male LUTS. https://uroweb.org/guideline/treatment-of-non-neurogenic-male-luts/#4. Accessed Jan 2021.

Administrative Problems

11

Faiz Motiwala, Hanif Motiwala,
and Sanchia S. Goonewardene

Administrative errors are a common source of complaints. They also form major contributor to medico-legal claims. Examples of these include:

- Failure to pass on important information
- Failure to arrange appointments, investigations or with appropriate degree of urgency
- Failure to review results of investigations
- Failure to arrange follow-up and or monitoring
- Mislabelling, misfiling and failure to check labels

Several of the cases discussed prior also fall into this category. One case in the 'Diagnostics' chapter, highlights inadequate review of the results of the investigations by the clinical team and poor feedback from radiology back to the team with the results of the investigation. Although there was an error in the diagnostics portion of management, the error can also be attributed to a failing of administration.

F. Motiwala
Queen Elizabeth Hospital, Woolwich, UK
e-mail: faiz.motiwala@nhs.net

H. Motiwala
Department of Urology, Southend University Hospital, Southend, UK

S. S. Goonewardene (✉)
Department of Urology, The Princess Alexandra Hospital, Harlow, UK

© The Author(s), under exclusive license to Springer Nature
Switzerland AG 2022
F. Motiwala et al. (eds.), *When Things Go Wrong In Urology*,
https://doi.org/10.1007/978-3-031-13658-0_11

11.1   The Referral

The first point of contact for a surgeon with a patient may be the referral letter of a GP. The letter should stipulate the problem at hand which is the responsibility of the GP. Following receipt of letter, it should be read promptly to ascertain and triage the urgency of the letter. The letter should then be dated and actioned as soon as possible. The surgeon is not responsible for the delays occurring prior to the receipt of the letter and dating the letter is proof of when one is able to action it. This can be important if there are substantial delays prior to receipt of the letter.

Often the letter will include relevant information strewn about, hidden in some paragraphs or even at the very end. It is important to avoid missing essential information which may surmise the reason for the referral such as painless frank haematuria! Fortunately, these patients are usually referred on the appropriate pathway though errors can still occur and patients can slip through the system. As such it is important to thoroughly read each letter lest any information be missed.

11.2   The Clinic Appointment

- Appropriate seniority
  - The patient seen in the clinic must be seen by someone of appropriate skill and seniority i.e. specialist registrar or above. A core surgical trainee may be appropriate provided they have the experience, or the means to discuss the case with the consultant prior to action or plans being formulated.
- Annual leave/sick leave
  - If one is due to be sick or away, consider the magnitude of leaving the clinic in the hands of an inexperienced or unsuitable junior. If there is no suitable alternative, it would be in everyone's best interest to cancel the clinic. While this may be disappointing for the patient, it would be safer than exposing both the unsuitable junior and the patient to each other.
- Active identification of patients
  - Patients should be identified actively rather than passively. Patients can mistake when their names have been called and there have been multiple instances where the wrong patient enters the consulting room and patient-sensitive data is provided to the wrong patient. The patient's name should be confirmed when they respond, in addition to a check of their date of birth and address. This also applies to checking correct investigations, results, and labelling samples correctly.
- The non-attender
  - A significant number of patients end up not attending their appointments, referred to as 'DNA's (did not attend/arrive). This may be applicable to clinic appointments as well as procedures or investigations. Many surgeons opt to write to the GP as opposed to patient, with a short sentence surmising 'Patient has failed to attend a third time. I will not be arranging a further follow up'. While it explains what has occurred to the GP it adds nothing to patient care.

The patient may have had valid reasons for not attending which have not been forwarded, or they fail to grasp the significance of their problem. These letters should be addressed to the patient, with the GP copied in. This will reduce delays in any diagnosis, the risk of complaints and most importantly, optimise care for the patients.

11.3   Requests and Investigation Results

Unfortunately, there is no clear system to allow systematic follow up of every request or investigation. There is the concern of the request or investigation being lost in the void that is the overburdened and stretched NHS service. In the service there are ways to reduce the burden with comments such as 'we will write with the result', only for the result to be lost or never acted upon as the results of the investigation may not arrive for weeks following the initial appointment. Numerous methods have been considered for appropriate follow-up of investigations and one should pick the one that best suits them, should they choose to use it. Some of these requests are automatically copy in the requesting consultant if there is a 'code-red' i.e. something which requires prompt action. The disadvantage of this is the need to rely on radiology both identifying and also reporting on the investigation. The result may also not be reported on for some time if it is a routine outpatient request.

One option is to have a book with a list of all pending investigations; these should be added to when one is requested and checked regularly. When the result is available, this can be signed off the results written to the patient/GP. This book could be shared among the outpatient department. Alternatively, there may be an online system or clinicians carry their own personal book or list of investigations to follow-up (with adequate data protection of course). Another option is to simply have a follow-up appointment of every patient after their investigation or a results clinic, but this places a stronger burden on the service to see patients, some of whom will not need more than simple reassurance that the results of their investigation are fine [1].

While there is a responsible consultant for each patient, the responsibility of these investigations should also lie with the requesting doctor. Juniors should be encouraged to take responsibility of following up investigations they have requested (or there should be an adequate follow-up system such as an MDT for histology results) and consultants should be informed of any investigations that have been requested, especially if the patient is discharged with pending results or awaiting an outpatient review. When juniors rotate, the follow-up of these investigations should also be handed over to the team, or the appropriate senior. If the patient is discharged from the ward there should be a clear follow-up plan of results indicated in the discharge letter.

Of relation, there are several documented cases in literature of retained or forgotten ureteric stents, with some having been forgotten for 10, or even up to 25 years [2, 3]. To this day there still do occur cases where patients have not been booked in for it despite there being a clearly documented plan for the removal of the stent. A forgotten stent is a 'never event' in the UK. These of course have the risk of ongoing pain or recurrent infections, and complications of encrustations, stone formation, stent fractures, hydronephrosis and even loss of renal function. Ultimately, improper follow-up of these brings upon patient morbidity, financial burden and increases the strain on existing resources. The use of stents across different specialties e.g. urology, interventional radiology, gynaecology etc. adds to the difficulty of monitoring these appropriately—for example, a patient with a gynaecological malignancy develops hydronephrosis secondary to compression from the mass—urology is consulted for their opinion and then a nephrostomy ± antegrade stent is requested to be performed by interventional radiology.

There needs to be adequate patient education and appropriate measures for follow-up. Some trusts have advocated the use of stent registers or a list of a manually entered database including patient details and when stent removal is required. However, these do require correct input of data and issues can occur with patient engagement or communication. Others have opted for the use of 'stent card' to improve patient education or even a 'stent tracker' application [4].

11.4   Discharge Plan

On discharge there should be a clear summary of the events—a couple of lines may be adequate for a patient who was admitted for a 1 or 2 days but a 6 week stay complicated by re-do operations, septicaemia and escalation to the Intensive Care Unit clearly requires a little more. The summary should also include a clear follow up plan. The ideal summary should mimic the ideal post-operative note with relevant details included. Such details should be communicated effectively to patients and allow them to engage more with their care. Pending investigations should be highlighted and a clear follow-up plan for these i.e. who will be doing it and when it should be expected. One should also remain sensible in their requests. Asking the GP to repeat urea and electrolytes in a patient in 1 week following recovery from an acute kidney injury (AKI) is an acceptable follow-up. Asking the GP to organise urodynamic studies and refer back to urology with the results is not acceptable. Be clever with the available facilities and don't shy away from reviewing patients sooner than the usual 6 weeks or 3 months—particularly if here had a tumultuous post-operative period and require a review sooner, perhaps within 2 weeks. Check local departmental policies and see what is available. For example, you may note yourself to be on-call and be able to ask the patient to come into the Surgical Assessment Unit or its equivalent for a review by yourself. If you are concerned, you owe to your patients.

References

1. Vermeir P, Vandijck D, Degroote S, et al. Communication in healthcare: a narrative review of the literature and practical recommendations. Int J Clin Pract. 2019;69(11):1257–67.
2. Kim DS, Lee SH. Huge encrusted ureteral stent forgotten for over 25 years: a case report. World J Clin Cases. 2020;8(23):6043–7.
3. Alex F, Lovin JM, Kelly EF, Connelly ZM, Nazih K. A 22-year-old retained ureteral stent: one of the oldest removed using a multimodal endourologic approach. J Endourol Case Rep. 2020;6:180–3.
4. Moghul M, Almpanis S. Stent cards: a simple solution for forgotten stents? BMJ Open Qual. 2019;8:e000612.

Prescribing

12

Faiz Motiwala, Hanif Motiwala,
and Sanchia S. Goonewardene

Prescribing medications is a common requirement for all clinicians. It is however prone to error and remains a dangerous area for any clinician. Junior doctors in particular can be at even greater risk due to an increased prescribing requirement while also having worked for fewer years.

Inadvertent prescribing errors form a significant portion of medical errors, despite being the most avoidable. English NHS organisations reported approximate 2.2 million incidents occurring between April 2019 to March 2020, with approximately 10% of these are medication errors [1]. The top three errors are wrong dosage, omitted/delayed drug administration and incorrect prescription or administration of drug. There errors can also arise from over-prescribing, incorrect transfer of medications, incorrect doses or spellings and not accounting for drug interactions or patient allergies. This of course only relates to those reported. A systematic review by Elliot et al., of which the data was originally published in 2018, estimated 237 million medication errors in one year (between 2015 and 2016), of which 28% were potentially clinically significant. Avoidable adverse drug events were estimated to have cost the NHS £98 million [2].

Four classes of drugs are associated with half of all preventable medication related hospital admissions; anticoagulants, e.g. warfarin or DOACs, antiplatelets, e.g. aspirin or clopidogrel, NSAIDs, e.g. diclofenac (commonly used to treat renal colic), and diuretics, e.g. furosemide [3]. The main adverse risk of the first three is

F. Motiwala (✉)
Queen Elizabeth Hospital, Woolwich, UK
e-mail: faiz.motiwala@nhs.net

H. Motiwala
Department of Urology, Southend University Hospital, Southend, UK

S. S. Goonewardene (✉)
Department of Urology, The Princess Alexandra Hospital, Harlow, UK

bleeding. When co-prescribing these medications, due care needs to be taken by prescribing the lowest safe dose or avoiding combinations where possible. Proton-pump inhibitors, e.g. omeprazole or lansoprazole should also be prescribed for gastric protection.

Even more dangerous are injectable medication errors, associated with harm or even death. A well-known case emerged in 2008 when a locum out of hours GP working his first shift, mistakenly prescribed 100 mg of diamorphine rather than 10 mg to a patient suffering from acute renal colic. The patient unfortunately died approximately 20 min after two intramuscular injections and the doctor was struck off by the GMC [4].

One UK study (EQUIP) found an error rate of 8.4% among all medication orders written by FY1s, with an error rate of 10.3% among FY2 doctors [5]. Other studies such as the PROTECT study similarly found error rates of 7.5% overall, with a higher error rate amongst FY2 doctors [6]. In particular, the majority of these were found to be made upon a patient's admission to hospital. Whilst the majority of these were detected early by the pharmacist before causing harm, unfortunately a few select cases still caused patient harm. These errors can arise from time-pressures in clerking patients or of the early morning ward round, lack of knowledge of the medication and appropriate dosage, unclear handwriting and mishearing the medication. At times when one is unsure, it is important to check with a colleague, senior or ward pharmacist. One should not be pressured to do anything beyond their competence, particularly if they have not heard of the medication or are not sure what it is. It is imperative to seek clarification in these circumstances. In situations where the junior is unaware of the medication, the senior clinician should assist them in the matter and view it as an opportunity for education.

Another aspect of prescribing is communicating to patients the indication for their medications. While some patients may lack the interest or capability to understand it, many will certainly take an interest in their own health. Explaining these medications including benefits, expected side effects or risks will foster both improved rapport and empower the patient in their own care. The patient will have a better understanding of what to do should they encounter issues and be able to discuss these more readily with the clinician with an understanding of it. If the patient has a basic understanding of common side effects, it can prevent unnecessary visits or discontinuation of their accord. Should the patient choose to discontinue a medication of their own choice, the clinician will have the knowledge that it is an informed choice and be able to work together with the patient to select a suitable alternative if possible.

It is essential to have a basic understanding of each medication prescribed and the reason behind it. The GMC advise you must only prescribe medications when you have adequate knowledge of patients' health requirements and that it serves their need [7].

Common medications in urology (though certainly not extensive) to be aware of include (Table 12.1) [8]:

The increasing elderly population with multiple complex co-morbidities such as atrial fibrillation, heart failure or previous strokes also poses challenge for their

Table 12.1 Common medication in urology: alpha-blockers, 5α reductase inhibitors, anti-cholinergics, mirabegron

Alpha-blockers
Indication: Benign prostatic enlargement
Mechanism: Antagonist of α-adrenergic receptors. Those prescribed for BPE target α-1 selective receptors. α-1 receptors in the prostate cause contraction of smooth muscle, thus α-1 blockers result in relaxation of smooth muscle.
Examples: Tamsulosin (Flomaxtra), alfuzocin (Xatral SR), prazosin (Minipress)
Common side effects: **Orthostatic hypotension**, nasal congestion, dizziness, lack of energy, headaches, drowsiness
5α Reductase inhibitors
Indication: Benign prostatic enlargement
Mechanism: Inhibits conversion of testosterone to dihydrotestosterone, i.e. prevents the formation of a more potent androgen, by inhibiting the function of the isoenzymes of 5α reductase. This serves to reduce the size of the prostate and improves lower urinary tract symptoms
Examples: Finasteride (Proscar), dutasteride (Avodart)
Common side effects: Loss of libido, erectile dysfunction, reduction in volume of ejaculate, infertility, gynacomastia, depression, anxiety, self-harm, dementia
Anti-cholinergics
Indication: Overactive bladder
Mechanism: Blocks the action of acetylcholine to its receptor in nerve cells—inhibiting parasympathetic impulses (involuntary contractions)
Examples: Oxybutynin (Ditropan), tolterodine (Detrusitol), solifenacin (vesicare)
Common side effects: Dry mouth, constipation, blurred vision, tachycardia, headache, **urinary retention, QT prolongation**
Mirabegron
Indication: Overactive bladder
Mechanism: Blockage of b3 adrenergic receptor
Common side effects: Arrythmias, constipation, diarrhoea, headaches, increased risk of urinary tract infections, nausea

management in the peri-operative period. The risk of the patient's venous thrombo-embolism or stroke needs to be balanced against their risk of significant bleeding which can make the procedure more technically challenging, result in hypovolae-mic shock, necessitate transfusions and increase the patient's morbidity and mortal-ity. Management of anti-coagulants (such as warfarin, direct oral anticoagulants (DOACs), heparin) or anti-platelets (such as clopidogrel or aspirin) in the peri-oper-ative period is essential knowledge for the surgeon.

Broadly, the four main options for managing patients on these medications include:

1. To stop these agents prior to surgery and restart some period after the surgery, e.g. TURP.
2. Continue through the surgical procedure, e.g. cystoscopy only.
3. Bridging therapy, e.g. low molecular weight heparin (LMWH) to balance the risk of bleeding vs. thrombosis.
4. To defer the surgery until these agents are not required.

Generally speaking, 5–7 days pre-operatively is an appropriate time to stop anti-platelet agents prior to surgery (though it may not be appropriate to stop in high risk patients), while timing for anti-coagulants varies. DOACs generally require 1–3 days and warfarin 3–5 days (with adequate bridging via LMWH for high-risk patients such as those with mechanical valves). Indirect thrombin inhibitors such as unfractionated heparin can require 12 h, LMWH between 12 and 24 h, and fondaparinux 24 h [9]. When stopped, these should be resumed when bleeding is no longer a serious risk (typically 4 days post-operatively though this can vary).

When the patient has anti-platelets or anti-coagulants stopped around an operation, the plan for their resumption should also be clearly documented in the post-operative note.

References

1. NHS England. NRLS national patient safety incident reports: commentary, Sept 2020. https://www.england.nhs.uk/publication/nrls-national-patient-safety-incident-reports-commentary-september-2020/. Accessed Jan 2021.
2. Elliott RA, Camacho E, Jankovic D, et al. Economic analysis of the prevalence and clinical and economic burden of medication error in England. BMJ Qual Saf. 2020;30:96–105.
3. Howard RL, Avery AJ, Slavenburg S, et al. Which drugs cause preventable admissions to hospital? A systematic review. Br J Clin Pharmacol. 2007;63(2):136–47.
4. GP Daniel Ubani struck off over fatal overdose. BBC News. https://www.bbc.co.uk/news/10349596. Accessed Mar 2020.
5. Dornan T, Ashcroft D, Heathfield H, et al. An in-depth investigation into causes of prescribing errors by foundation trainees in relation to their medical education: EQUIP study. 2009. Final report to the General Medical Council. http://www.gmc-uk.org/FINAL_Report_prevalence_and_causes_of_prescribing_errors.pdf_28935150.pdf. Accessed Mar 2020.
6. Ryan C, Ross S, Davey P, et al. Prevalence and causes of prescribing errors: the PRescribing Outcomes for Trainee Doctors Engaged in Clinical Training (PROTECT) study. PLoS One. 2014;9(1):e79802.
7. General Medical Council. Good practice in prescribing and managing medicines and devices. https://www.gmc-uk.org/ethical-guidance/ethical-guidance-for-doctors/prescribing-and-managing-medicines-and-devices. Accessed Mar 2020.
8. British National Formulary. https://bnf.nice.org.uk/. Accessed Mar 2020.
9. Tikkinen KAO, Cartwright R, Gould MK, et al. EAU guidelines on thromboprophylaxis in urological surgery. https://uroweb.org/guideline/thromboprophylaxis/. Accessed May 2021.

Diagnostics

13

Faiz Motiwala, Hanif Motiwala,
and Sanchia S. Goonewardene

Diagnostic tests are an essential component of medicine. Furthermore, some diagnostic tests allow for intervention. Diagnostics comprise of several components. Within urology, several investigations are commonly used and a good understanding of these will facilitate both optimal care for the patient and reduce the probability of medico-legal problems arising.

- Clinical Examination including digital rectal exam and testicular exam
- Bedside tests, e.g. urinalysis
- Blood tests including tumour markers such as prostate specific antigen (PSA)
- Imaging, e.g. X-ray, Computer Tomography (CT), Magnetic Resonance Imaging (MRI), intravenous pyelography, voiding cystourethrogram, retrograde urethrogram
- Nuclear medicine, e.g. PET scanning, renal scintigraphy
- Urodynamic studies, e.g. cystometry, uroflowmetry, pressure-flow studies, urethral pressure profile, leak point pressure, post-void residual volumes, electromyelograms (EMG)
- Endoscopy, e.g. cystoscopy, ureteroscopy
- Histopathology, e.g. cytology, histology

Each of these needs to be approached in a critical logical manner. It is important to understand the relevance of each investigation to the appropriate pathology. Appropriate application of these will facilitate optimal management of patients

F. Motiwala
Queen Elizabeth Hospital, Woolwich, UK
e-mail: faiz.motiwala@nhs.net

H. Motiwala
Department of Urology, Southend University Hospital, Southend, UK

S. S. Goonewardene (✉)
Department of Urology, The Princess Alexandra Hospital, Harlow, UK

© The Author(s), under exclusive license to Springer Nature
Switzerland AG 2022
F. Motiwala et al. (eds.), *When Things Go Wrong In Urology*,
https://doi.org/10.1007/978-3-031-13658-0_13

while preserving costs. While the majority is guideline and evidence based, some tips will come from personal experience or teaching from seniors. An important aspect of diagnostic tests is the correct balance in the investigation of disorders. Under-investigation may lead to inappropriate diagnosis or inadequate management, whereas over-investigation exposes the patient to excessive testing and unnecessary costs.

One facet of over-investigation has been the emergence of 'defensive medicine'; the process of investigation to protect oneself from medico-legal problems arising. By ensuring the investigation has excluded something, clinicians rest easy with the knowledge the patient is indeed safe from a particular condition and consequently the clinician is also safe from any medico-legal issues. This can lead to the performance of unnecessary investigations. A clinician needs to consider the ramification of each investigation performed. Was the blood test penetrating the patient with a needle necessary? Was the radiation exposed to the patient from the X-ray or CT scan justified? Will these change the management plan of the patient, or make any impact upon the patient?

13.1   Case 1: An Unnecessary Operation

A 56-year-old male with no significant past medical history was referred by his GP to a urologist due to elevated PSA and abnormal findings on digital rectal exam. This was confirmed by the consultant in the clinic and following several investigations, the patient was eventually booked for elective radical prostatectomy for prostate cancer. A junior registrar later requested a pre-operative chest X-ray though there was no clear indication or reason as to why they had done so. The consultant was not aware of the investigation as the junior colleague did not inform him of it.

The patient underwent radical prostatectomy; he suffered post-operatively with erectile dysfunction but was otherwise clinically well and discharged from hospital. 6 months later the patient deteriorated clinically and was admitted to hospital. Investigations confirmed an advanced primary lung cancer, unsuitable for treatment beyond palliation. On review of his previous imaging, a shadowy lesion was identified and reported on the previous chest X-ray performed pre-operatively. The patient sued for clinical negligence and the performance of an unnecessary operation. The case was settled in court with a moderate sum pay-out.

13.1.1 Appropriate Investigation and Follow Up of Results

This case highlights several issues in the care of the patient. Firstly, the patient underwent an unnecessary investigation. A pre-operative chest X-ray is not indicated in a patient of this age and without co-morbidities or symptoms. In effect, the identification of such a lesion was by pure chance. While the test identified a lesion in this case, it does not justify performing such a test routinely. Secondly, there was no follow-up by the team of the investigation. The registrar failed to inform the consultant that the investigation was requested, nor did he follow up the results. Thirdly, the radiologist who reported the investigation did not flag the lesion as a code red or inform the clinical team of the results. This may be understandable if there are a lack of symptoms or indications given in performing the X-ray, however this patient was due to have a radical prostatectomy performed for a known diagnosis of prostate cancer. Consequently, the patient underwent an operation which may have been avoided had the clinical team followed up on their initial investigation. Further investigation may have been performed sooner and the metastases caught sooner. This operation also resulted in a poorer quality of life as he was sexually active prior to his operation.

An essential element of performing an investigation lies in appropriate follow-up of said investigation. The requestor of the investigation should take responsibility in the follow-up of the investigation. If a junior is requesting on behalf of a responsible consultant; the consultant should be aware of the investigation being performed and the results copied to them. This is especially important for outpatient investigations, or investigations requested to be performed as an outpatient following discharge from hospital. These should be highlighted in the discharge letter, and both the GP and patient should be aware of the follow-up following this investigation, e.g. whether there is a follow-up clinic, a phone call with results or follow up in the community. Without these appropriate measures, the risk of these being lost without adequate follow-up is high. It is expected that investigations as an inpatient are performed promptly and followed up by the appropriate ward team with good handover where required.

13.2   Case 2: Missed Prostate Cancer

A 45-year-old male presented to his GP for respiratory problems. He had multiple investigations performed including a test for prostate specific antigen (PSA). The PSA was elevated at 4.1; this was highlighted in the documentation and noted for discussion in the following meeting. The patient was not informed of the result. The patient was seen by another doctor at the practice and no further action was taken. The patient presented again 2 years later with back pain. The patient was referred however was not initially under the 2 week wait scheme adding a slight further delay to their management. Investigation confirmed an elevated PSA of 100 and they went further to have confirmation of a metastatic biopsy proven prostate cancer. The patient filed for medical negligence and the case could not be defended.

13.2.1 Appropriate Follow Up of Patients and Handover Between Clinicians

This case highlights several learning points. It can be devastating to everyone involved to miss a potential early cancer diagnosis at a much more treatable stage. While unclear as to why the GP decided to order a PSA test, the result came back abnormal, and this should have been actioned. It emphasises the need to not only follow-up an investigation, but to perform appropriate handover and act upon results. The initial physician did not choose to repeat the PSA, perform a digital rectal exam to confirm or exclude a diagnosis of prostate cancer, nor did they inform the patient of the abnormal result. They should have made a 2 week wait referral at this stage. Furthermore, there was inadequate handover with the second physician not following up on the investigation either. Most importantly, the patient should be informed of the diagnosis and the result; this may have allowed for the patient to also initiate a follow-up sooner if required to provide treatment [1].

13.3   Case 3: A Missed Testicular Torsion

A 20-year-old male presented to the Accident and Emergency Department with a 6-h history right testicular pain with associated nausea and vomiting. The testicle was noted to be normal size and lie, with mild swelling. The patient also reported that the pain had mildly improved from onset though this pain did persist as did his nausea. The patient was reviewed by urology SHO who had documented their findings including an intact cremasteric reflex but was unsure about the diagnosis and wanted to exclude torsion. The patient was booked for and underwent an urgent ultrasound scan which was reported as an epididymitis. The SHO had discussed their findings with the urology registrar however the patient was never reviewed by the registrar, with the team agreeing upon the likely diagnosis of epididymo-orchitis due to the ultrasound findings. The patient was advised it may take some time for the pain to settle, but to wear his scrotal support and complete his course of antibiotics. The patient's pain continued for 3 days before he felt it was unbearable and returned to the Emergency Department. He was re-referred to urology and reviewed by the registrar who noted significant swelling and scrotum discolouration and booked the patient promptly for surgical exploration. Intra-operatively a necrotic testicle was identified, and the patient underwent right orchidectomy with three-point fixation of the left testicle. A review of the ultrasound noted there was likely reduced flow to the testicle and the testicle was still potentially salvageable at the time. The patient filed a claim that the diagnosis should have been made on the first visit with potential salvage of his testicle. He was instead subject to significant ongoing pain and a traumatic event that significantly affected his mental health and future.

13.3.1 Diagnostic Evaluation with Ultrasound

A meta-analysis published in 2019 by Ota et al. [2] analysed 2116 patients across 26 studies and determined the overall diagnostic sensitivity of ultrasound for testicular torsion was 0.94 (95% CI 0.83–0.98), and pooled specificity was 0.98 (95% CI 0.94–1.00). Studies after 2010 showed sensitivity of 0.95 (95% CI 0.84–0.99) and specificity of 0.98 (95% CI 0.93–0.99). It should however be noted that ultrasound is highly operator dependant and high-resolution ultrasound is not widely available. It is often not possible to perform an ultrasound within the time critical stage of the presentation, with testicular salvage rates >90% only if performed within 6 h of onset of pain. This is further complicated by how ischaemic damage is dependent upon degree of torsion, type of torsion and completeness of vascular occlusion. Ultrasound scan alone is also not sufficient to exclude a testicular torsion and should be corroborated with a clinical examination, preferably by someone with adequate clinical experience. It is a tool which can strongly support a clinical diagnosis however should not be solely relied upon, particularly in a time sensitive situation! In these circumstances when there is suspicion for torsion, the patient should proceed immediately for surgical exploration unless the patient himself declines and voices a concern for operative exploration. In these cases, the patient should be re-assured and the risks of delaying an exploration should be clearly explained with clear documentation of the discussion.

13.3.2 Clinical Suspicion and Surgical Experience

A missed or delayed presentation of testicular torsion can be difficult for all those involved. Testicular torsion can potentially present similarly to epididymitis. Cases of testicular torsion have been noted to present with gradual onset discomfort and cases of epididymitis present with sudden onset pain. Presence or absence of cremasteric reflexes, scrotal oedema, (transverse) lie of the testis, tenderness along the testicle or epididymis, Prehn's sign (relief upon the examiner lifting the testicle) can guide the clinician to a diagnosis but are not definitive.

The patient should ideally have been examined by a more senior or experienced enough member of the team. When there is a genuine suspicion, there should be low threshold to explore the testes intra-operatively instead of booking the patient for and relying on an ultrasound scan. Negative findings in a scrotal exploration are a much more reassuring finding than to wait for an ultrasound scan that confirms a dying or dead testicle. That is not to say that every testicle should be explored as that would clearly be inappropriate. A careful history and examination typically do guide one between an epididymo-orchitis or testicular torsion. With this in mind, you should also be open to the potential diagnosis of intermittent testicular torsion progressing to infarction. This can also fool imaging findings. If there is doubt about the diagnosis, the patient should be reviewed by someone with adequate experience and if doubt remains, it is much safer to explore.

References

1. Mottet N, Cornford P, van den Bergh RCN, et al. EAU guidelines on prostate cancer. https://uroweb.org/guideline/prostate-cancer/. Accessed Jan 2021.
2. Ota K, Fukui K, Oba K, Shimoda A, Oka M, Ota K, Sakaue M, Takasu A. The role of ultrasound imaging in adult patients with testicular torsion: a systematic review and meta-analysis. J Med Ultrason (2001). 2019;46(3):325–34.

Operating Theatre Issues

14

Faiz Motiwala, Hanif Motiwala,
and Sanchia S. Goonewardene

The operating room is a breeding ground of potential errors. These errors can give rise to unexpected post-operative complications which may result in litigation. Ironically these cases of litigation are more likely to occur following a 'routine' case as opposed to a complex case in which due precautions and meticulous planning have taken place.

Some of the serious errors that can occur in the operating room include:

- Incorrect patient
- Performing an operation on the wrong site
- Performing the wrong operation
- Inappropriate surgical sterilisation
- Leaving improper surgical materials inside the patient's body
- Errors in anaesthesia
- Injury to organs/vessels/nerves/tendons with inappropriate detection or management of these
- Neglect in monitoring patient vitals or correction of these intra-operatively
- Inappropriate management of venous thromboprophylaxis or antibiotic prophylaxis

A well-known case is of Mr. Reeves, who underwent a routine nephrectomy with drastic consequences. What was to be a routine right nephrectomy ended in disaster

F. Motiwala
Queen Elizabeth Hospital, Woolwich, UK
e-mail: faiz.motiwala@nhs.net

H. Motiwala
Department of Urology, Southend University Hospital, Southend, UK

S. S. Goonewardene (✉)
Department of Urology, The Princess Alexandra Hospital, Harlow, UK

© The Author(s), under exclusive license to Springer Nature
Switzerland AG 2022
F. Motiwala et al. (eds.), *When Things Go Wrong In Urology*,
https://doi.org/10.1007/978-3-031-13658-0_14

85

when the left healthy kidney was removed in error. The discovery of the mistake was too late to return the kidney and a further operation was attempted to restore function to the chronically diseased right kidney. This was however unsuccessful, and he was placed on dialysis, eventually succumbing to septicaemia and passing away 5 weeks following his initial operation [1].

There were several failings which occurred leading up to the serious error. The registrar performing the operation had made an incorrect entry into the Urology Department using information from a wrongly completed admission slip. On the morning of the surgery, during ward round he did not speak to the patient as the patient was asleep. The operating registrar was informed by a medical student who had discerned that the incorrect kidney was being removed. She noted this on the X-ray as well. However, her concerns were dismissed. The consultant in charge also made the error of placing the X-ray back-to-front which resulted in the positioning of the left nephrectomy. He had also failed to consult his registrar on the matter.

These problems could have been prevented, through discussion with the patient on the morning of the operation, comparison of the planned operation to the notes/consent form and consultation between the registrar and consultant on the planned operation. The use of technology and computers also removes a factor of human error in placing the X-ray incorrectly, but this should always be checked nonetheless as there can be errors in labelling or uploading the X-ray image. This case also raises the issue of hierarchy, communication and teamwork. Had the registrar simply listened to the student raising her concerns, such a grievous error could have been prevented. However, hierarchy can remain as a barrier to something this simple even in the current climate. Juniors should be encouraged to speak up if they feel there to be a problem at *any* stage.

Surprisingly, wrong site surgery is not an uncommon error, with a total number of 226 wrong site surgeries (48% of all never events), reported in NHS hospitals in the period of 1st April 2019 to 31st March 2020 [2]. It is consistently one of the commonest "never events" to occur in UK hospitals since data collection began in 2009. These errors do not impact purely on the life of the patient but can have long-lasting impacts on the surgical team, affecting both their mental status and working capacity. Factors that have been identified as potential contributory factors include [3, 4]:

1. Booking documents not verified by office schedulers
2. Schedulers accepting verbal requests for surgical bookings instead of written documents
3. Unapproved abbreviations, cross-outs, and illegible handwriting used on the booking form.

Some of these factors are less common with the usage of online booking request forms, however it is a reminder of the importance of avoiding abbreviations and particularly avoiding handwriting 'R' for right or 'L' for left—there are many individuals whose R's and L's can be mistaken for another.

There has been the introduction of several safety checklists to combat errors such as this, most notably the WHO checklist which serves to increase communication and teamwork to reduce the number of errors or adverse events. The checklist has been shown by Haynes et al. to reduce in-hospital complications from 11% to 7% and reduce death rates from 1.5% to 0.8% [5]. Trusts within the UK utilise the previously known National Patient Safety Agency (NPSA)'s adapted version of the WHO Surgical Safety Checklist, published as the 'Five Steps to Safer Surgery' in 2010: consisting of briefing, sign-in, time-out, sign-out and debriefing [6]. Below is a summary of the process including the timing and what is carried out within each step (local practice may vary from trust to trust and this is a generalisation) (Table 14.1).

Some people may view it as simply a tick-box exercise to complete and commence with the surgeries, which is exactly what it can devolve to if the team view it simply as that, significantly contributing to the risk of a 'never event' occurring.

The responsibility of the briefing falls to the surgeon and as such should be prepared to lead it. The anaesthetist should also lead and discuss any issues from their review. The team briefings are there to facilitate discussion and ensure errors beyond simply the wrong operation/wrong site operation, including the various aspects that are highlighted above. The briefing especially allows for correct order of patients, ensuring that the equipment is there prior to induction of anaesthesia, and best practice is followed for the patient within the peri-operative period.

Concerns regarding the briefing include the length of operating time lost and rallying the relevant team members for the brief. This should however not deter an essential process which serves to reduce the risk of errors and optimise patient care. The issue of rallying team members relates more to an organisational issue and the

Table 14.1 Five steps to safer surgery

Five steps to safer surgery	Timing	Procedure
1. Briefing	• At the beginning of a list, or when staff change	• Introduction of team members/roles • Order of patient list • Anaesthetic or surgical concerns
2. Sign-in	• Prior to induction of anaesthesia	• Confirmation of patient/operation/consent form • Allergies • Airway concerns • Equipment check
3. Timeout	• Prior to start of surgery	• Ensure above is correct • Check of VTE prophylaxis, warming, glycaemic control, antibiotics
4. Sign-out	• At the end of the operation • Prior to staff leaving operating theatre	• Confirm correct procedure • Swab/instrument count • Specimen correctly labelled • Equipment issues • Post-operative management
5. Debriefing	• At the end of the list	• Evaluation of list/day • Learning from incidents • Remedy of problems

briefing should occur either as soon as possible or be set to occur at a specific time, e.g. at 08:15 following patient reviews by both surgeon and anaesthetist and when theatre staff are available. The concern of operating time lost is a fallacy; the process takes a few minutes and should be used to discuss concerns with patient anaesthetic, ensure correct equipment is available for the operation and plan the order of the list (which may differ owing to updated information or administrative errors in booking the list). Booking errors may also have occurred resulting in listing of incorrect operations which can be highlighted in the briefing.

Patient-relevant factors to be aware of include:

- Foreign body/metalwork—stent, joint replacement, pacemaker, valve, graft
- Anti-platelets, e.g. aspirin, clopidogrel or anti-coagulants, e.g. DOAC or warfarin
- Precautions—present or previous MRSA infection, hepatitis, HIV
- High-risk of variant-CJD, e.g. previous corneal transplant, neurosurgical dural treatment, human growth hormone treatment
- Relevant investigations—these should include up to date urine microscopy samples or relevant imaging, e.g. a CT Urogram or staging CT scan prior to the operation.

These should be identified within the pre-assessment stage either during clerking or during the anaesthetic assessment.

The introduction of the team is also more than just a tick-box; it facilitates appropriate communication and acts to reduce hierarchal barriers. The team should feel comfortable expressing concerns and be able to contribute. This is similarly so with the debriefing; this may occur prior to lunch or at the end of the day when people are vying to leave and is often overlooked or glossed over. A debrief is important to review the cases of the day and highlight any concerns from staff such as equipment problems or something that could have been done differently or improved. In most cases there will be little to discuss but it is especially important when a serious event has occurred. This event may be when a surgeon is under due stress and lose their temper with a staff member, barking orders or communicating in a way that may be viewed as blunt or rude. There may be a near-miss due to equipment problems or poor organisation. In these circumstances a debrief is important to reflect, discuss what happened, check on theatre staff members and apologise if appropriate.

14.1 Intra-operative Equipment

For operations to run smoothly, equipment must be working to a good quality standard. This includes basic monitoring equipment, diathermy pads, surgical tools, irrigation and suction, in addition to more specific equipment such as X-rays, laser machine, the da Vinci robot or various tools such as cystoscope, ureteroscope and other adjuncts to the procedures. Required equipment should be ordered and organised well in advance of the operating day. Concerns with any equipment should be highlighted in the team briefing or discussed in the sign-out of the relevant case or debrief at the end of the list.

Keeping equipment in the back of the room or in a separate room, away from the patient until the completion of the surgical time-out can avoid team-members from becoming distracted or pre-occupied with the set-up of the instruments.

14.2   Intra-operative Communication

Communication between staff during an operation is essential. The surgeon needs to be clear as to what they want from their scrub nurse or team and avoid demanding, unreasonable requests or shouting. Music can be a good mood-setter (provided everyone tolerates your taste!) and can help you to stay calm or work more efficiently, but it shouldn't be too loud as it can end up serving as a distraction or if it needs someone to raise their voice to communicate in the room. Most people find that it does help them relax (though it certainly would depend on the type of music), and it has been found to improve cognitive function of listeners, improve mood, and create a sense of well-being [7, 8]. If it is interfering with communication or there is a stressful moment that you or the operating surgeon wants silence for, it might however be sensible to stop it at that moment.

14.3   Perioperative Complications

Complications can arise from any operation, and these should be explained to the patient in due detail prior to the operation, with all alternatives including no treatment offered to the patient. Should a complication arise within the procedure, it is the duty of the responsible clinician to inform the patient.

Common sources of complaints in urology include [9]:

- Vasectomy
- Circumcision
- Prostate cancer—TURP
- Nephrectomy
- Ureteroscopy
- Percutaneous nephrolithotomy
- Cystostomy

14.4   Theatre Organisation

It is important to highlight lapses in theatre organisation can also impact on patient care and management. Especially in this time of the COVID pandemic, there are often staff shortages with most services being overworked. Theatre efficiency must also be maintained to allow prompt treatment of patients. Part of this is having a well-motivated team and leadership from the top, with a role model being set for the whole team. It is important that if any member of the theatre team do have concerns, they are listened to and their issues addressed. It is also important to make sure when a patient is listed for theatre, that it is the appropriate operation and that it is listed for the correct amount of time. It is also important to make sure that it is for the correct list, with the correct equipment available.

14.5   Surgical Emergencies

There will arise situations (particularly late evening/night-time), in which a patient needs to go to the operating room, such as a testicular torsion, but the Emergency CEPOD anaesthetist is already in the middle of a procedure. The anaesthetist and theatre co-ordinator/staff should be informed clearly of the emergency case, for example that there is an urgent exploration of testis required as it may otherwise infarct. On occasion they may say that there will be a delay of even several hours for the current case to finish or to wait your turn, which is not acceptable. A second anaesthetist (which may be the anaesthetic consultant on call) should be called in and a second operating theatre opened. The case should be thoroughly explained to the theatre staff and anaesthetist to appreciate the urgency of the situation, with clear documentation of this in the notes. If needed, do *everything* you can to get the second operating theatre opened.

References

1. Dyer O. Doctors suspended for removing wrong kidney. BMJ. 2004;328(7434):246.
2. NHS resolution: never events data. https://www.england.nhs.uk/patient-safety/never-events-data/. Accessed Mar 2020.
3. Devine J, Chutkan N, Norvell DC, Dettori JR. Avoiding wrong site surgery: a systematic review. Spine (Phila Pa 1976). 2010;35(9 Suppl):S28–36.
4. The Joint Commission Center for Transforming Healthcare. The wrong site surgery project. 2011.
5. Haynes AB, Weiser TG, Berry WR, et al. A surgical safety checklist to reduce morbidity and mortality in a global population. N Engl J Med. 2009;360(5):491–9.
6. National Patient Safety Agency. 'How to guide'. Five steps to safer surgery. London: NPSA; 2010.
7. Faraj AA, Wright AP, Haneef JH, Jones A. Listen while you work? The attitude of healthcare professionals to music in the operating theatre. J Perioper Pract. 2014;24(9):199–204.
8. Weldon SM, Korkiakangas T, Bezemer J, Kneebone R. Music and communication in the operating theatre. J Adv Nurs. 2015;71(12):2763–74.
9. Osman N, Collins G. Urological litigation in the UK National Health Service (NHS): an analysis of 14 years of successful claims. BJU Int. 2011;108(2):162–5.

Human Factors in Healthcare

15

Faiz Motiwala, Hanif Motiwala, and Sanchia S. Goonewardene

Human factors, or 'ergonomics', play an extensive role in healthcare delivered to patients. There are a multitude of identifiable factors which can be optimised. It is the responsibility of the clinician to raise their own concerns or problems, but it is also important for colleagues to be mindful of each other and if a genuine concern is noted, it is their duty to act upon it.

It is defined as [1]:

Enhancing clinical performance through an understanding of the effects of teamwork, tasks, equipment, workspace, culture and organisation on human behaviour and abilities and application of that knowledge in clinical settings.

The principles of Human Factors focus on optimising human performance through an improved understanding of the individual, interactions between individuals and their interactions with the environment. Human factors have been extensively studied in other industries, notably the aviation industry. They have studied human-factors rule through accident analyses, the black-box, and simulator-research. Studies have identified that between 60% and 80% of incidents were caused by teamwork-failure (consisting of human factors, chain of errors and human performance limitation) [2]. Like aviation, human errors in medicine can be disastrous with grave consequences.

Cognitive psychologists commonly divide errors emerging from human factors into [3]:

F. Motiwala
Queen Elizabeth Hospital, Woolwich, UK
e-mail: faiz.motiwala@nhs.net

H. Motiwala
Department of Urology, Southend University Hospital, Southend, UK

S. S. Goonewardene (✉)
Department of Urology, The Princess Alexandra Hospital, Harlow, UK

© The Author(s), under exclusive license to Springer Nature
Switzerland AG 2022
F. Motiwala et al. (eds.), *When Things Go Wrong In Urology*,
https://doi.org/10.1007/978-3-031-13658-0_15

- Skill-based errors i.e. slips and lapses. These may be due to factors affecting the cognitive state such as fatigue. These are unintended actions.
- Mistakes—decision making errors. This is an intended action which generates a problem occurring due to lack of knowledge or an incomplete understanding of the situation.

There is a third type of error known as violations. These are *intentional* failures and will not be discussed.

A slip arises from intrusions when thinking about something else e.g. another patient you are worried about or the next difficult case. These tend to happen with familiar tasks. Lapses arise from memory failures, particularly in tasks which are complex or have multiple steps.

The medical field is particularly susceptible to errors in human factors for several reasons. Doctors work long shifts and can be highly understaffed in some locations. While medicine and perceptions continue to evolve and improve, traditional views may still permeate in some areas. These include hierarchies which may forms barriers to communication, seniors not accepting input from junior members, or differing perceptions of teamwork among team members. Surgical trainees may experience further demands in the modern era with reduced theatre time, the need to be present for the purpose of improving their skills, or in following the examples of their seniors. This can be worsened by the presence of a 'blame culture' whereby one fears speaking out, accepting mistakes or taking responsibility lest they receive criticism, retribution or worse.

Factors that may affect the cognitive function of a doctor include:

- Fatigue
- Depression
- Burnout
- Morale
- Knowledge and skills
- Tools and equipment
- Support
- Pressure
- Time of day
- Environment
- Technology/computers

There are also organisational factors affecting human performance:

- Organisational structure
- Management of others
- Provision of equipment
- Maintenance of equipment
- Training and selection
- Scheduling
- Communication

These factors can increase the risks of errors and mistakes happening. A doctor may find themselves falling asleep during work owing to a culmination of fatigue. At least two junior doctors have died in car crashes following night shifts since 2011. One study conducted by the Association of Anaesthetists of Great Britain and Ireland and published in *Anaesthesia*, received 2170 responses from UK Anaesthetic trainees. Of these, 84% of respondents felt that they were too tired to drive home after a night shift and 57% said that they had experienced a crash or near miss in doing so [4]. The infamous case of the wrong kidney being removed was greatly influenced by human factors.

Doctors have higher rates of mental illness in comparison to the rest of the population and some professional groups. In the UK it is estimated that 10–20% of doctors become depressed at some point during their career [5]; this figure is also likely an underrepresentation owing to the nature of the condition and barriers they may face from concerns of social stigma. A doctor's drive for success, commitment to their work and perfectionism may put them at an even increased risk of mental health problems.

'Burnout' is a term to describe emotional and mental exhaustion following repeated exposure to stressors. While there is no strict definition, it relates to several symptoms consisting of exhaustion with or without physical symptoms, alienation from work and emotional distancing, and ultimately a reduction in performance where they may be difficulty in concentration. Some experts feel it may be driven by other mental health disorders such as depression or anxiety, and vice-versa. These factors in combination with the environment may contribute to poor morale. With these expectations and risk of either burnout or mental health problems, it is extremely important for doctors to monitor their status and health. There can however be huge difficulty in even identifying or reflecting on what one's current situation is, let alone then having the strength to come forward with it for fear of social stigmatisation. There needs to be increased support in place, particularly for new doctors acclimatising to new environments or areas. These situations may in fact even be long-standing and people who have enabled unsustainable practices to continue, certainly with an overhaul in the entire system needed for these.

It is essential for there to be a supportive culture, and for errors to be identified and lessons drawn from these cases to improve patient safety (via a root-cause analysis). Increased reporting should be encouraged with a move away from the blame-culture. A system-based approach to error investigation is much more relevant to the NHS and considers the organisational problems leading up to the error.

A surgeon is not infallible, and slips, lapses or mistakes can occur. These may occur in any setting and are not limited to within the operating theatre. It can occur on the ward, in the outpatient setting, or even when you are at home receiving a phone call about a patient. As with any complications, it is one's duty to inform the patient of an error that has occured. In the post-operative phase this should be done when the effects of the anaesthetic have worn well-off that the patient would be able to recall the event. You should not shy away from the prospect of an apology. A sincere and frank apology will aid in restoring trust between the patient and clinician to allow future care to occur, while also reducing the chance of a complaint or litigation being filed.

A common misconception is that an apology is an admission of guilt or liability. Section 2 of the Compensation Act 2006 [6] stipulates: 'An apology, an offer of treatment or other redress, shall not of itself amount to an admittance of negligence or breach of statutory duty.' Rather, an apology acknowledges that something potentially could have been improved. Acknowledgement is the first step in reflection and learning, to ultimately take further steps to prevent it from happening again.

References

1. Catchpole. 2010. Cited in Department of Health Human Factors Reference Group interim report. National Quality Board, 1 Mar 2012.
2. Sexton JB, Thomas EJ, Helmreich RL. Error, stress, and teamwork in medicine and aviation: cross sectional surveys. BMJ. 2000;320(7237):745–9.
3. Jhugursing M, Dimmock V, Mulchandani H. Error and root cause analysis. BJA Educ. 2017;17(10):323–33.
4. Rimmer A. Over half of anaesthetic trainees have had car crash or near miss after night shift, survey finds. BMJ. 2017;358:j3328.
5. Brooks S, Gerada C, Chalder T. Review of literature on the mental health of doctors: are specialist services needed? J Ment Health. 2011;20(2):146–56.
6. Compensation Act 2006, Chapter 29, p. 3. https://www.legislation.gov.uk/ukpga/2006/29/part/3. Accessed Jun 2020.

Managing Difficult Seniors

16

Sanchia S. Goonewardene, Hanif Motiwala,
and Faiz Motiwala

Teams in medicine and more specifically surgery, must always be a cohesive unit. It is therefore difficult, when you are in a situation where the person you are meant to be guided or trained by is not on your side.

16.1 Managing Direct Conflict

One of the more startling things as a junior registrar, was when my AES blurted out, 'people who have been registrars for a while, are difficult to train as they are set in their ways', within the first month of the job. Reflecting on this comment as an older registrar, it is important to highlight that whilst waiting for my NTN, I had completed a number of fellow positions, but they did not provide any training requirement. I had to highlight to my consultant that I am there as an ST4 trainee and needed training to develop and improve. Another comment made was, 'you have been registrar for a number of years, but not thought how to improve your knowledge of the field'. In theatre 1 day, on three separate occasions, one of the senior team had taken out my jugular three different times. The next week, I had written an op note on which the feedback was good. The next op note written was even better, but the same thing happened again. The lesson is, always keep your cool and judgement in high pressure situations. Always remain focused on your objective no matter what. Never take your eye off the ball, which is to be trained, no matter how

S. S. Goonewardene (✉)
Department of Urology, The Princess Alexandra Hospital, Harlow, UK

H. Motiwala
Department of Urology, Southend University Hospital, Southend, UK

F. Motiwala
Queen Elizabeth Hospital, Woolwich, UK
e-mail: Faiz.Motiwala@nhs.net

95

many times your jugular is taken out. It can happen several times in a week. The key is to develop resilience and to keep your goals in mind. A little bit of tolerance will go a long way. The goal is to be the best you can.

16.2 Being a Female in Medicine

During my time as a junior registrar a formal complaint that had been raised against me by a senior nursing sister on the ward. There were two issues to address: My hair not being tied up and my attitude towards some nurses on the ward. I had previously been spoken to about my hair not being tied up from a consultant, which had been re-iterated at my mini ARCP. The day in question, my hair had been tied up and then came down. During the course of the day, I tend not to look in a mirror. The first time I was told off about my hair, I was sharply told to 'tie up my hair'. The second time this happened, I was taken to a room alone and screamed at. Unbeknownst to me, not long after this incident my consultant was told about my hair and a DATIX was filled in and submitted. These instances are frequent in any field of medicine. The key is to find people who support you through it. Fortunately, as I get on well with other ward nurses, theatre nurses and the specialist urology nurses, they all kindly showed me great support. Indeed, the urology specialist nurses took me on an online shopping spree to buy hair accessories. It is important to be mindful that hair being tied up is important as part of infection control, which is critical to ensuring the best possible care for patients.

Being a female in medicine, can often be littered with conflict. The key is to have female mentors who support you as part of a group reflection. As I work in a male dominated field, being firm and decisive can be mistaken as being condescending or even arrogant, when all you are trying to do is be clear, precise, and concise when managing patients, to ensure optimal care and safety.

The key to getting through issues like this is to rally more support from the team you work with (nursing and medical). For all of us as a team to look at the whole picture and try to find solutions together, will help to ensure the best atmosphere for the care of our patients. This will also result in improving our communication so that we can work better together, as 'Teamwork definitely makes the dreamwork'. This will be a recurrent theme throughout my career. As a girl in medicine, expect to have to work twice as hard as you will be judged not just on clinical skills, but other attributes and personality. If we can improve our communication skills, we will improve our teamwork. This can be done within a supportive team environment, both from medical and nursing staff. In this way we can ensure safer and better patient care, as well as empowering each other to become better and stronger.

16.3 Fixed and Growth Mindsets in Medicine

To understand what has happened over the past 6 months, it is important to understand the two differences between Professor Carol Dweck's fixed and growth mindsets. This significantly impacts on teaching, leadership, and management. A fixed mindset means that if you fail, it is eternal, and you are forever labelled as this.

Google specifically has labs set up for employees to fail. The lesson is to see what they can learn from failure. The culture of fixed mindset teaching must change as this significantly impacts trainees. When you encounter such a style in a trainee or trainer, it is not constructive. You should aim to have a growth mindset. The growth mindset is a desire to learn. Therefore, intelligence can be developed, criticism can be learnt from, lessons can be gained from others, you can persist in the face of setbacks, and your effort leads to mastery.

During my training, my desire to learn has been demonstrated by taking on board what consultants have said, from going to MPS courses, going on a communications presentation lesson, internal reflection by completing a 360, and even doing a hostage negotiation course.

To change from a fixed to growth mindsets, there are several steps. The first step is to constantly evaluate yourself. By using WBAs you can constantly assess yourself. With a growth mindset, you accept you can fail. The next step is to recognise fixed and growth mindsets exist. A fixed mindset is a choice. Feedback, which is given in a belittling or humiliating way, is as good as no feedback at all, and actually has destructive abilities as has been identified here. The lesson is keep going and persist, with all the learning outcome goals to change opinions from a fixed mindset to a growth mindset.

16.4   What to Do when Training Fails

There are several components needed for successful training. As trainees and trainers, we should aim to have a growth mindset. We want to grow and learn. According to Maslow, this includes an awareness of self, self-esteem, and a safe environment. Within that comes trust, belonging, and an awareness of when an environment is difficult. It is important for trainers not to create an unsafe environment with no element of trust or belonging. According to the work done on 'Flow' the optimal performance occurs when challenge and skill go hand in hand. The problem is, when these two are out of sync. This creates not a learning environment, but an environment in which there is panic, terror and where you cannot learn or retain information. This kind of environment would also go against Kolbs four stages of learning.

In a protected 'safe' environment, you can just grow and grow. At Watford, this environment is not provided, certainly for the first 6 months. As a result, the level of growth has not been comparable. The other factor that comes into play is group dynamic, the work of Tuckman. This includes different steps such as forming, storming, norming, performing, adjoining. A smooth transition between stages, results in better performance.

Leadership in Medicine

17

Sanchia S. Goonewardene, Hanif Motiwala, and Faiz Motiwala

17.1 Development of Leadership Under Pressure

Central to the values of Surgery, are leadership skills. This involves not just being part of a team, but also leading a team. Surgery is by definition a high-pressure job. By sharing a vision of what is expected from team members, engaging the team and setting clear expectations, managing and supporting performance, it allows opportunities for development and take steps to develop those team members further.

17.2 Leadership Styles in Medicine

In today's NHS, flexibility and adaptability are composite requirements for any practicing clinician. By having flexibility between different styles, any clinician can adapt to almost any scenario. Autocratic and distributed leadership would apply to theatre teams and ward rounds, where the whole team would chip in. Bureaucratic leadership applies to teaching and training, sticking to the rules. Paternalistic leadership often applies to training juniors. The only style that does not apply in medicine, is the Laissez- faire- the hands-off approach. This does not work in surgery. I have had situations where I needed support and instead been told 'you are on your own'. A surgical team is a supportive team, not an individual alone.

S. S. Goonewardene (✉)
Department of Urology, The Princess Alexandra Hospital, Harlow, UK

H. Motiwala
Department of Urology, Southend University Hospital, Southend, UK

F. Motiwala
Queen Elizabeth Hospital, Woolwich, UK
e-mail: Faiz.Motiwala@nhs.net

© The Author(s), under exclusive license to Springer Nature Switzerland AG 2022
F. Motiwala et al. (eds.), *When Things Go Wrong In Urology*, https://doi.org/10.1007/978-3-031-13658-0_17

99

17.3   Coaching and Mentoring as Part of Leadership

Coaching and mentoring forms a core part of urological training. A robust structured educational approach is needed. For quick decisions, a mentoring role is often easier, however, when relating this to juniors, it may not always make them independent. In the long run, we want them independent and thinking on their feet. In these cases, a coaching approach is often easier.

17.4   A Supportive Leader Can also Be a Supportive Team Player

I once received a phone call from one of the consultants asking where I was as everyone mentioned I was on call. That day I was not in hospital as I was not rota'd on call. I was able to tell the consultant on call who was on call that day. I then forwarded him a copy of the rota, with a message that if no registrar turns up, to give me a call and I will come in. I called him at 0900. He had managed to get hold of the on-call team. On reflection, it is really important that patient safety is maintained, and colleagues feel supported. This makes a big difference to all team members involved. When I reflected on how this would be from the consultant's perspective—it is very difficult to cover an on call singlehandedly, especially in a busy job. Were this to happen, patient safety would be compromised, and that is something that cannot be allowed to happen.

17.5   Good Leadership Is Built on Trust

Trust is built on sincerity, consistency, competence, reliability, commitment and integrity. Good rapport is the key to building good relationships, whether it be going for coffee together or having lunches with any member of staff. Trust is a valuable commodity which must be built over time.

Managing a Complaint

18

Faiz Motiwala, Hanif Motiwala,
and Sanchia S. Goonewardene

There are a myriad of potential sources of errors and complaints, as well as how to prevent them. Despite these implementations, one may find themselves at the receiving end of a complaint. This is the risk every professional face in their lifetime at least once during their career. You may be accused of negligence where an outcome was poor but due to no fault of any member. The important thing to do is to remain calm and remember that you are not alone in this. We will discuss the general proceedings and what to expect should you find yourself in this situation.

18.1 The Complaints Procedure in the NHS

This follows the NHS and social care complaints procedure, introduced in England on first April 2009. It is governed by the Local Authority Social Services and National Health Service Complaints (England) Regulations 2009 [1]. It obliges NHS organisations to have arrangements in place to handle patient complaints (Fig. 18.1).

Complaints may be made to all NHS bodies or providers of NHS healthcare (including commissioning bodies and primary care) and may be directed at the organisation or the individual providing the service. Many complaints ae resolved at this stage with local investigation and resolution. If the complaint is unhappy with the response from an organisation or individual, they can ask the Ombudsman to

F. Motiwala
Queen Elizabeth Hospital, Woolwich, UK
e-mail: Faiz.Motiwala@nhs.net

H. Motiwala
Department of Urology, Southend University Hospital, Southend, UK

S. S. Goonewardene (✉)
Department of Urology, The Princess Alexandra Hospital, Harlow, UK

© The Author(s), under exclusive license to Springer Nature
Switzerland AG 2022
F. Motiwala et al. (eds.), *When Things Go Wrong In Urology*,
https://doi.org/10.1007/978-3-031-13658-0_18

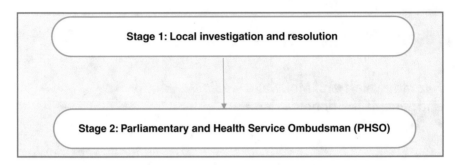

Fig. 18.1 The NHS complaints procedure

review the complaint. Similarly, if the receiver of the complaint is unhappy about the response from the organisation, they can also ask the Ombudsman to review [2].

The MDU report from their experience that patients who do complain seek one or more of the following: a thorough investigation with an explanation of what happened and why, assurance it will not happen again and a sincere apology [1]. Remember, a sincere apology is powerful and in the UK is not an admission of liability [3]. Patients are entitled to a prompt, sympathetic, open, constructive, and honest response; this should also not adversely affect the care provided to the patient and is reflected in GMC's Good Medical Practice (Paragraph 31) [4].

A complaint may be made within 12 months of the subject matter being complained about or 12 months after the date which the subject matter of the complaint came to be noticed by the complainant. There are however exceptions which may be considered if there were good reasons for the complaint not being made within the timeframe and if it is possible to still investigate the complaint effectively and fairly.

18.2 Responding to the Complaint

Within the NHS, it is unlikely that you would have to write the complete response to the complaint yourself as this is typically done by the complaints manager. You may have to however provide an account of what happened to aid the written response or even meet with the complainant for discussion. Alternatively, you may not be the subject of the complaint, but involved in the investigation and response, or providing independent clinical advice.

The complaints made be made through several means:

- In person
- Telephone
- Email
- Letter

All of these must be acknowledged within 3 days by the responsible body. The exception to this is oral complaints that can be resolved to the complainant's satisfaction within 1 working day of being received. This is important to bear in mind if you are aware of this or have been told directly and can work to resolve this, for example if the patient tells you in person on the ward or within the clinic setting. If it is simple and you can resolve this with patient satisfaction, a written response is not required. It is however good practice to document the discussion and keep it for your records. The MDU advise that this is done in a complaint file, separate from clinical records.

Following receipt of this complaint, discuss it with your line manager and begin formulating a plan for the response as soon as possible. Be open-minded and flexible in your approach. Take it with seriousness. There is always a lesson to be learnt.

Within the body of the complaint, you should be able to identify what concerns the patient is raising and what they are requesting. It should also allow you to identify potential problems to be corrected. Sometimes these issues may arise from a misunderstanding and a simple explanation in a colloquial language should be used to clarify these issues.

A planned response requires a thorough investigation and review of the records. This is where clear detailed documentation is essential to corroborate memory, from the exact date and time of events, to who was involved at which step in the care of the patient. What were the differentials? What were the negative findings? Was there appropriate consent? Who else was present during the round or clinic appointment? Who was the chaperone? In these situations, you need to state which aspects of your account are based on memory, notes or from usual practice. It may be that you recall the event but note a lack of documentation regarding a particular matter. Quoting from memory is perfectly acceptable and if the details of the event escape you, what you would do in usual practice. Under no circumstances is it acceptable to alter these documents. If the records have been amended then it needs to be clearly marked, dated, and signed.

The letter of your account should preferably be typed (for legibility) and written in first person e.g., instead of 'Mrs X was examined on…', to write 'I examined Mrs. X on…'. Not only does this clarify to the reader the involvement of the responder but shows a more active and positive approach to dealing with the problem at hand. The body of the letter should include:

- Your identity and rank e.g., Consultant, registrar and if locum
- A detailed report with a chronological description event including relevant medical history, working diagnosis/diagnoses, investigations/reports and treatment performed
- A response to each concern highlighted by the patient.
- If the complaint is addressed to multiple clinicians, only comment on the part of the case you were involved in. It is not appropriate to comment or provide opinions on the acts or omissions of other colleagues unless they are under your supervision.
- An analysis of the complaint—identification of the concerns and an action plan to remedy the situation

- Simple explanations for technical terms, including drugs and what they are used for. Or what a procedure such as 'nephrectomy' i.e., removal of kidney means.
- Medical terms written fully (no acronyms)
- Enclosure of a copy of the physical notes. If some written portions are unclear, a typed transcript to accompany these notes.
- An apology where appropriate

This response should be written promptly—ideally as soon as possible though within 6 months. Regulations specify that the complainant should be updated and informed of the reasons for the time taken in writing if there is no response within 6 months.

Most complaints are fortunately resolved successfully at the first stage. A good response will require time and thought, and you will thank yourself for with your thorough documentation and keeping to good medical practice.

References

1. NHS complaints: local investigation and resolution. The MDU. 2017. https://www.themdu. com/guidance-and-advice/guides/nhs-complaints-local-resolution Accessed Sept 2020.
2. NHS Complaints Guidance. Department of Health and Social Care. https://www.gov.uk/gov-ernment/publications/the-nhs-constitution-for-england/how-do-i-give-feedback-or-make-a-complaint-about-an-nhs-service. Accessed June 2020.
3. Compensation Act 2006 Chapter 29 Page 3. https://www.legislation.gov.uk/ukpga/2006/29/part/3. Accessed June 2020.
4. General Medical Council. The duties of a doctor registered with the General Medical Council. 2013. www.gmc-uk.org/guidance/good_medical_practice/duties_of_a_doctor.asp. Accessed June 2020.

The Anatomy of Failure and How to Avoid It

19

Paul Tiller

19.1 An Introduction to Failure

"Insanity: doing the same thing over and over again and expecting different results"—Unknown.

Has there even been an occasion in your life when you failed at something you tried?

I hope the answer is a resounding Yes! If not, then perhaps you are not quite ready for this chapter. The reality of life is that we all fail on an almost constant basis.

Consider an infant who is looking to take their first steps, do they just jump up and get going? Well, no, it's a wobble to their feet and usually falling over again quite quickly. The key thing here is what do they do next? Is it an endless cycle of repeating the process and getting the same outcome time after time, or do they adjust, tweak, or change something in their approach?

A mentor of mine once said to me, "In life, statistically we will get more things wrong than we do right, and that's okay. Without this ratio, how would the book-making or stockbroking industries be viable?" On the surface, this may seem a glib statement, but there is a lot of truth in it. Not getting it right on every occasion is very normal, to be expected even. However, it's only by studying the concept of failure in more depth do we discover that there is a process that lies hidden within and it's the ignorance of this that leads to true repeated failure.

Consider when you have started something new, perhaps a job, relationship, business, or hobby. Think about the excitement that you felt as you began this. You knew what to do, how to do it, what was next and were excited by it all, right? But

P. Tiller (✉)
Chartered Institute of Personnel and Development (CIPD), London, UK
e-mail: paul.tiller@wecandu.co.uk

F. Motiwala et al. (eds.), *When Things Go Wrong In Urology*,
https://doi.org/10.1007/978-3-031-13658-0_19

then what? After a while, did something get in the way? Did you stop doing the things that you know were going to keep you on that path? Did you avoid it? It's surprisingly common. In fact, there are no end of ways that we can find to avoid doing what's necessary—and if we are experienced procrastinators, we excel in finding these!

Once we realise that we are no longer doing what we need to do, we start to feel bad. But it's okay, as we can normalise this through the creation of excuses. Think about your most common excuse that you may use about why something did not get done. "I didn't have the time" is the most common one. Is this on your list?

Excuses are a great accelerant of failure and once we are adept at using them, things come crashing down to earth fast and failure becomes inevitable. Is it our fault? Of course not! We then expend even more energy on blaming anything and anyone that we can. "It's the government", "It's the economy", "It's the boss", or "It's…whatever". Feel free to insert your own blame statement here.

So, we are back to square one, yet the "insane", as described above, take great delight in repeating the process, again and again, often knowingly. I'm sure you know someone who's life is littered with multiple starts and restarts, initiative after initiative after initiative, only for them all to end in failure and doom (Fig. 19.1).

Let's revisit our infant trying to stand up and walk. Whilst they cannot express the process above, it's the same for them as it is for us. They will try to stand up, stop doing something that will allow them to succeed, fall to the floor and look around with bemusement. We know from experience that they eventually succeed. So, what do they do next?

The answer is as relevant to the infant as it is for us. They **learn** from the experience and **change** what they are doing. Perhaps they grab hold of a nearby chair or table to help them stay upright. Perhaps they spend more time perfecting crawling first. Whatever it is, something different is attempted that will allow them to progress. Do they fail again at the task of standing? Probably. But this new failure, at a different point in the process, will lead to further insight and therefore progress towards their goal of walking will be made.

The key to the small but significant change is that they have taken responsibility, consciously or unconsciously, for creating a different outcome. Is it not time for you to do the same?

Fig. 19.1 The cycle of failure

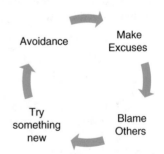

19.2   Creating the Case for Change

"Failure should be our teacher, not our undertaker. Failure is delay, not defeat. It is a temporary detour, not a dead end. Failure is something we can avoid only by saying nothing, doing nothing, and being nothing."—Denis Waitley

Reconsidering the failure process above, it always starts with avoidance. The wilful sabotage of our own path to success that takes us off course. So how can create the case for success within ourselves?

There are four key success factors for sustained change. Let's examine them in turn.

19.2.1 Do I Have Clear Goals?

The biggest reason for avoiding the things you need to do to be successful is simply not knowing where success lies. Very few people set their lives up with written, structured, and meaningful goals.

Even then, simply having goals is no guarantee of success. There are some qualifying factors that we need to address.

- The goals need to be compatible with you and your core beliefs.
- The goals must be of the required quality, clarity and be underpinned with a clear purpose and provision of benefit for others.
- The goals need to be sufficiently challenging but not unattainable. They need to avoid the trap of being too easy, or a different kind of avoidance can overtake us, as comfort, boredom, and lethargy creep in.

This is supported by the effect of challenging goals and feedback in relation to task performance [1] which supported hypotheses regarding the effect of goal setting on an individual's performance, if accompanied by either specific process or specific outcome feedback. The highest measured performance was recorded for participants who had **specific, challenging goals, supported by specific process and outcome feedback**.

When set up correctly, high quality, meaningful goals are one of the most powerful tools you can possess. When you focus on these daily, you get into a rhythm of action and activity as you move towards them. With this pattern of repeated action and application of change into your life, you will become a performance and achievement machine.

19.2.2 Am I Sufficiently Focused?

Even the best goals are rendered useless if not supported by a relentless focus and action on our part. *"Weak and scattered thoughts are weak and scattered forces. Strong and concentrated thoughts are strong and concentrated forces."* [2].

Without making changes to our ways of working and aligning ourselves to an action centred mindset, we seriously hamper our chances of achieving our goals. We are unclear about what we want to be, to have, want or do. Only by having great goals coupled with a clear commitment and daily focus on them do we build our personal power.

19.2.3 Do I Have a Clear Action Plan?

"No matter how small the improvement, we're going to do it and create a culture of continuous improvement", [3]

To further support the first success factors, a clear plan of action is required, a plan that breaks down your goals into manageable units. Break the overarching goals that you have set into smaller, major tasks. Beneath this, work out and list the activities that you need to perform every day. These small individual steps are the elements that you need to keep you active and moving towards the bigger goal.

If you wanted to learn a new language, you could break this down into learning a new word or phrase every day. You wouldn't become fluent overnight obviously, but with repeated practice could become highly proficient over time. Every activity that you want to consider for a goal can be broken down in this way. The key to success is to document the steps, your actions and progression every day. Performance athletes make small changes to their effort, style, or approach constantly, these so-called marginal gains are small in nature, perhaps only 1% of the overall game but, when applied repeatedly, have been recognised with some of the greatest performers and performances in modern sport.

19.3   Have I Overcome My Mental Barriers?

So now we know what we need to do to become successful, why isn't it the case that we just get on and do it? After all, we have explored and rationalised all the reasons that is keeping us from continuing a successful course of action.

The answer lies in two small words. **Mental barriers**.

Take a few moments now to be honest with yourself and think about what mental barriers regularly come up for you. Make a note of them to the side. The list may be short or long, but we **all** have them regardless of who we are.

Here are some of the most common mental barriers that I see regularly in my practice:

1. Fear
2. Doubt
3. Worry for the future
4. Lack of confidence
5. Fear of being successful

Do you recognise any or many of these in yourself? This short list quickly breaks out into more detail once we think about it further. What is driving our thinking in this way? Where did we learn to adopt and accept these mental barriers as part of our everyday life?

The answer can be found in our past, as we have picked these up along life's journey thus far. Our previous experiences, our upbringing, our families, our friends, our workmates and from those people whom we look up to and respect, will all contribute to our mental barriers in some way. These are learned, subtly and sub-consciously over many years or decade. These, left unchecked, will prevent you from fulfilling your ambition, no matter how well you set this up in other areas of your life.

Our mental barriers are manifested in small ways. These can be negative thoughts, repeated performance of knowingly poor decisions or, by the voice in your ear that draws you back from making that bold decision or enacting a major change for the better.

19.4   Plotting a Course for Success

"The secret of change is to focus all your energy not on fighting the old, but on building the new",
—Socrates

The reason that we are here is that we haven't set things up properly for ourselves or within ourselves. We need to reconsider both our long-term aiming points and our short-term approaches to progress and achievement. We can create a strong foundation for this by applying the four key principles that I have already mentioned.

1. Set great goals
2. Develop a laser focus
3. Create a comprehensive plan of action
4. Identify and tackle any mental barriers

It is entirely possible to you to undertake the above and I encourage you to do so right away. Just by doing these things, you will already be well ahead of most other people on this planet. However, it can be a lonely journey if undertaken alone and the opportunities to engage in avoidance behaviours loom large. After all, who is going to be there to hold you accountable for your outcomes? It's surprisingly easy to award yourself a free pass!

In the Goals Research Study [4], three key impacts of increasing attention to goals and how they are formulated, managed, and held accountable for are noted.

1. **The positive effect of written goals was supported:** Those who wrote their goals accomplished significantly more than those who did not write their goals.
2. **There was support for the role of public commitment**: those who sent their commitments to a friend accomplished significantly more than those who wrote action commitments or did not write their goals.

3. **The positive effect of accountability was supported:** those who sent weekly progress reports to their friend accomplished significantly more than those who had unwritten goals, wrote their goals, formulated action commitments, or sent those action commitments to a friend.

This research indicates that with the provision of the right support, your chances of achieving the goals you set are significantly improved. It should come as no surprise then that those who truly seek to lock in their path to success, engage with a professional coach and/or mentor.

19.5   What Is Coaching and Mentoring?

Coaching and mentoring are very effective approaches to developing yourself. Both have grown in popularity, with many choosing to utilise the services of a coach or mentor to enhance their skills, knowledge and performance based around their goals.

Here I offer a definition of coaching and mentoring, distinguishing between the two and emphasise the need to link with overall learning needs. It looks at those typically responsible for coaching and how to develop a coaching mindset. Deciding when coaching is the best development intervention is key to harnessing its potential.

There remains a lack of understanding about how best to use coaching and mentoring—for instance, the situations in which it will be most effective. The figure below (Fig. 19.2) considers this in 2 axes—timeframe and level of direction (ask vs. tell).

Fig. 19.2 The ask and tell axes for coaching and mentoring

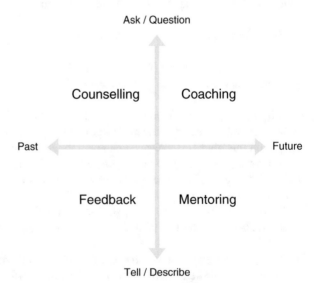

We will examine coaching and mentoring in more detail presently. It must be noted that counselling is another dimension that requires the intervention and support of a professionally qualified specialist and is to be kept separate from this discussion. Feedback, however, is an important part of our professional and personal experiences and is often the stimulus for you to seek a coaching and mentoring intervention.

19.6 Coaching

"A good coach can change an outcome. A great coach can change a life"—John Wooden

Coaching aims to produce optimal performance and improvement. It focuses on your specific skills and goals, although it may also have an impact on your personal attributes such as social interaction or confidence. The process can last for a defined period, but more often forms the basis of an on-going support relationship. There are some generally agreed characteristics of coaching:

1. It's a non-directive form of personal development in that actions and outputs are co-created by you and your coach.
2. It focuses on improving your performance and developing you as an individual.
3. The coach becomes your accountability partner.
4. It provides you with the opportunity to better assess your strengths as well as your development areas.
5. It's a skilled activity, which should only be delivered by people who are trained to do so.

19.7 European Mentoring and Coaching Council (EMCC) Definition of Coaching

To provide an industry view, the EMCC defines coaching as thus:

"It is a professionally guided process that inspires clients to maximise their personal and professional potential. It is a structured, purposeful, and transformational process, helping clients to see and test alternative ways for improvement of competence, decision making and enhancement of quality of life."

19.8 Mentoring

Mentoring describes a relationship in which an experienced person shares their knowledge to support you in your development. It calls on the skills of questioning, listening, clarifying, and reframing that are also associated with coaching.

112

P. Tiller

Mentoring relationships work best when they move beyond the directive approach of a senior colleague 'telling you it how its is', to one where mentor and mentee both learn from each other. An effective mentoring relationship is a learning opportunity for both parties, encouraging sharing and learning across generations, roles and even professions.

The outcome of successful mentoring is development of skill and capability of the person being mentored.

19.9 European Mentoring and Coaching Council (EMCC) Definition of Mentoring

To provide an industry view, the EMCC defines mentoring thus:

"A developmental process, which may in some forms involve a transfer of skill or knowledge from a more experienced person to a less experienced, through learning, dialogue and role modelling."

19.10 Roles and Responsibilities within the Coaching and Mentoring Process

There are responsibilities to consider for all the roles in the coaching and mentoring process, whether as a practitioner or participant. The figure below, outlines these (Fig. 19.3).

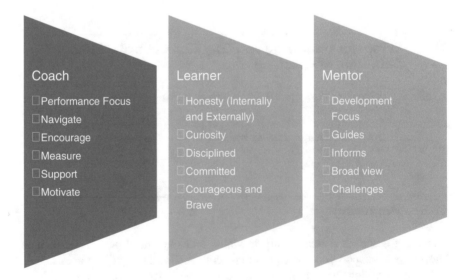

Fig. 19.3 The behaviours required of each role in a coaching or mentoring arrangement

19.11 The Benefits of Having a Coach in Your Life

Now that we have explored the anatomy of failure and introduced the notion of coaching and mentoring as a supporting resource, what are the real-world benefits to you for having your own coach.

Consider that most, if not all, high performing people in business and sport interact with one or more coaches several times a day. This work is purely focussed on the actions in the now and how they will move them towards a better future.

A coach will help you to find and form the goals that have real power. Goals that you will be able to consider every day and motivate you to work towards them. It's a sad fact that very few people set their lives up in this way, where they intrinsically understand what they want to have, be, do or become. Few have taken the time to set up a series of manageable actions and activities that will form their unique development journey.

A tiny fraction of us wakes up each day with these at the forefront of our minds. There are a small number however, who are so self-aware that as they awake, they sit bolt upright in their beds and say to themselves, "I have so much to accomplish today, and I know what I have to do next". Although we are all, theoretically, capable of achieving this state of self-actualizing, most of us will not do so, or only to a limited degree. In his Hierarchy of Needs, Maslow (1970) estimated that only 2% of people would reach this state of self-actualization.

The reality is that essentially most people don't change from a repeated journey through the anatomy of failure, but the beautiful thing about human beings is that **we can**. We can look within ourselves and make changes, but it requires an element of discipline, a solid sense of direction, an application, and a coach to help you through the process.

I encourage you to be curious about where you are today, what has brought you here but, more importantly, where is it that you want to be? Having a coach alongside you will make a significant different to your approach and outcomes in your life.

References

1. Christopher Earley P, Northcroft GB, Lee C, Lituchy TR. Impact of process and outcome feedback on the relation of goal setting to task performance. Acad Manag J. 1990;33(1):87–105.
2. Kehoe J, Banks R. Mind power into the 21st century. Bc Zoetic Inc: North Vancouver; 2017.
3. Sir Dave Brailsford—the 1% factor. 2016. https://youtu.be/NQxYlu12ji8. Accessed 19 June 2021.
4. Matthews G. Goals research summary. Dominican.edu; 2021. https://www.dominican.edu/sites/default/files/2020-02/gailmatthews-harvard-goals-researchsummary.pdf. Accessed 29 June 2021.

Raising a Concern in Training

20

Sanchia S. Goonewardene, Hanif Motiwala, and Faiz Motiwala

20.1 General Medical Council Duties of a Doctor

Training is often a difficult path to negotiate. If trainees have concerns during training, this can also be difficult to manage, as no one wants to be labelled as a trouble-maker. According to the General Medical Council Code of Conduct, patient safety is key, and under the duties of a doctor, also include maintaining patient safety and raising a concern through appropriate channels (Good medical practice (paragraph 25). Concerns include patient safety issues, unsafe working conditions, inadequate training, bullying, or fraud allegations.

20.2 Raising a Concern in Training

As a trainee, the first port of call is within the department. Speak to an educational supervisor. If you feel you can't approach them, speak to a clinical supervisor. Should that fail, try the clinical lead. If none of them are responsive and you still have concerns, approach the Director of Medical Education. Should this not work, then approach the training programme director firstly, and then your postgraduate dean. Alternatively, the BMA are present as a defence organisation, and MPS/MDU relating to clinical work.

S. S. Goonewardene (✉)
Department of Urology, The Princess Alexandra Hospital, Harlow, UK

H. Motiwala
Department of Urology, Southend University Hospital, Southend, UK

F. Motiwala
Queen Elizabeth Hospital, Woolwich, UK
e-mail: Faiz.Motiwala@nhs.net

20.3 Reporting

Using the DATIX reporting system, both clinicians and non-clinicians can report a wide variety of concerns; not just patient safety concerns, but also attitude and behaviour. It is important that information is documented concisely, precisely and prospectively if required, so it is all up to date, factual and accurate. It is important that the clinical lead and management staff are aware of the situation, and both listen and investigate it appropriately, with outcomes from DATIXs' being presented at clinical governance meetings. It is important to reflect and develop as part of medical practice. The GMC has guidance on raising and acting on concerns (Fig. 20.1).

It is critical that when any incident happens, the reporting is kept factual, and it is reported to the relevant authority. Professionalism must be always maintained, and when going through a period of difficulty, a mentor is often a great source of help and support.

Fig. 20.1 Adapted from GMC guidance on raising and acting on concerns

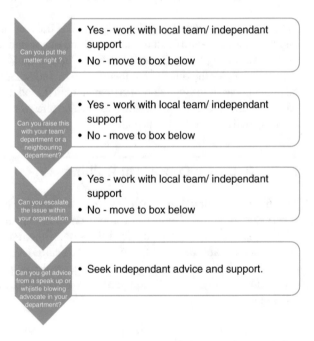

The GMC Investigation

21

Faiz Motiwala, Hanif Motiwala,
and Sanchia S. Goonewardene

An investigation may arise for numerous reasons. Several thousand concerns are raised with the GMC annually and these are triaged to the response required. From the information gathered they may: immediately progress to investigation, have a provisional enquiry, be referred to the employer/responsible body, or closed without further action. Approximately 80% of these are closed either as they do not relate to a doctor's fitness to practice or are matters that cannot be investigated [1].

1. The Provisional Enquiry
2. The Full Investigation

21.1 The Provisional Enquiry

If the GMC do choose to investigate, they may contact you with a letter and the initial step of the investigation may begin—the provisional inquiry [2]. It can be a terrifying experience for anyone to receive this letter but does not carry a deeper significance or a measure of your inability as a doctor. These are mere basic inquiries to formulate a view on the doctor's ability to practice. It is not a full investigation. They are quick (63 days) and do not require substantial information or evidence, as opposed to a full GMC investigation over 6–12 months. The advent of these provisional enquiries in 2014 has prevented many cases requiring a full

F. Motiwala
Queen Elizabeth Hospital, London, UK
e-mail: Faiz.Motiwala@nhs.net

H. Motiwala
Department of Urology, Southend University Hospital, Southend-on-Sea, UK

S. S. Goonewardene (✉)
Department of Urology, The Princess Alexandra Hospital, Harlow, UK

© The Author(s), under exclusive license to Springer Nature
Switzerland AG 2022
F. Motiwala et al. (eds.), *When Things Go Wrong In Urology*,
https://doi.org/10.1007/978-3-031-13658-0_21

investigation; in 2017 alone a total of 614 provisional enquiries were begun, with 391 closed (63.7%) saving these doctors the burden and stress of a full investigation. Had these not undergone a provisional enquiry, there would have been a total of 1920 full investigations as opposed to 1529.

Contact your medical defence organisation (such as the MDU or MPS) for support. Complete any basic paperwork such as employment details form if requested and return this to the GMC. Do not reply or comment unnecessarily to the GMC (except for the employment details form) until you have sought support from your medical defence organisation or equivalent.

Typically, the GMC may obtain a statement from a witness or request an expert opinion to explore the concerns raised. The evidence is obtained by a GMC case officer upon which the GMC form a decision. This evidence may arise from a variety of sources including reports and medical notes/documentation. If you are aware of certain documentation or notes that would be required or beneficial, identify them and request them early to obtain them within the timeframe of the provisional enquiry.

At this stage you can submit a reply, but this should be done with the utmost care. In our experience, doctors can damage their own case by phoning the GMC or making inappropriate replies or comments. Saying too much or writing something which suggests a lack of insight can raise concerns with the GMC. Stay calm. Discuss with any colleagues you are comfortable in discussing the matter with. Seek the support of your medical defence organisation. Gather the relevant documents. Reflect on the case, such as using the approach to the ethical dilemma algorithm or through whatever means you find easiest. If you have written this case in your portfolio or discussed it at your appraisal, these should also be reviewed and reflected upon. Liase with your medical defence organisation and with their advice, form a clear response. The submitted documents should follow a clear structure and be indexed; a summary of the contents page keeps the information organised.

21.2   The Investigation

The provisional enquiry may not provide enough information to form a decision and the GMC may then proceed to the full investigation. You should not be immediately alarmed if this is the case; many of these investigations end with no action.

The reasons for opening an investigation may include:

- Misconduct
- Poor performance
- A criminal conviction or caution
- Physical or mental health resulting in an inability to practice medicine
- Insufficient knowledge of English

Often the concerns that result in investigation arise not from knowledge or technical skills, but rather their professional practice and behaviour, such as whether the doctor listens to patients, respects patient confidentiality, treat their staff members well etc.

Being pro-active and constructive in response to allegations are viewed more positively than those that are dismissive or fail to address the matter at hand.

References

1. Fitness to practice statistics 2017. GMC. https://www.gmc-uk.org/-/media/documents/fitness-to-practise-statistics-report-2017_pdf-76024327.pdf. Accessed March 2020.
2. Our investigation process. GMC. https://www.gmc-uk.org/concerns/information-for-doctors-under-investigation/how-we-investigate-concerns/our-investigation-process.   Accessed March 2020.

Approach to GMC Investigations, How to Handle Them and What to Do

22

Patrice Wellesley-Cole, Maurice Cohen, Charlie Easmon, and Jonathan Makanjuola

> *Reputation of the profession is more important than the fortunes of any individual member. Membership of a profession brings many benefits, but that is part of the price.*
> —Lord Bingham MR in Bolton v Law Society 1994 61 WLR 512, often cited in regulatory proceedings.

The medical profession has a privileged and trusted role in society; in return they are required to live up to their professional standards. This carries with it responsibilities. But what happens if a doctor becomes the subject of a General Medical Council (GMC) investigation? How does he/she handle it and what should they do?

A doctor facing such an investigation should be prepared by being legally represented and a member of the British Medical Association (BMA), their trade union which will give them both financial and moral support, which is vital at such a stressful period in their careers.

All doctors are mandated to pay the GMC annual retention fees and other registration fees which have changed since April 2008. The GMC is a registered charity in England and Wales. Its aim is to—

> *protect patients and improve medical education and practice in the UK by setting standards for students and doctors. We support them in achieving and exceeding those standards and take action when they are not met.*

P. Wellesley-Cole (✉) · M. Cohen
St. Hugh's College, Oxford, UK

C. Easmon
International Association of Physicians for the Overseas Services (IAPOS), London, UK
e-mail: charlie@yourexcellenthealth.com

J. Makanjuola
Department of Urology, King's College Hospital, London, UK

The purpose of this chapter is to situate the GMC in a legal context and provide a critical analysis of its value as a means of providing doctors with a fair hearing in the context of Diversity, equity and inclusion (DEI).

22.1   Initial Consideration and Referral Allegation

At the beginning of the investigation, the GMC will inform a doctor of any complaints in writing, in stages, averaging over 12 months [1, 2]. Multiple streams of reporting to the GMC include the Trust (their employer), a patient or colleague. If a Trust reports a doctor, there will be an internal investigation first.

Misconduct, deficient professional performance, fitness to practise, criminal convictions or cautions and not having the required English language skills are all within their remit.

1. They will request comments (unless it's a self-referral).
2. Request key information to close the investigation as soon as practicable, for example employment details.
3. Contact your medical defence union, usually the BMA/British Medical Association.
4. They will also consider practically whether you should be suspended immediately or your practice restricted. In such cases it will be referred to the Medical Practitioners Tribunal service (MPTS) currently headed by Judge David Pearl for interim orders. Interim orders are provisional, not final measures sought during proceedings before a hearing or trial.

For example, if concerns received relate to convictions or decisions from another regulatory body, the GMC can refer doctors to the MPTS, but will not do them for minor offences such as parking.

22.2   Before the Hearing

Observing such an investigation first is advisable as GMC hearings are open to the public, unless in camera. A full conference with one's lawyer is also necessary as the GMC often have Queen's Counsel (QCs) to represent them. They may serve expert opinions which for either side may say if actions were negligent, explicable or explainable compared to the competence of an average doctor in their specialisation.

The pre-hearing process covers documentary evidence such as medical records, witness statements, expert reports and assessment of health, English and performance which may lead to a referral to the MPTS for such interim orders.

22.3 The Hearing

Your case file with all the statements, reports and relevant evidence will be before the Investigatory Panel who will have familiarised themselves with the material facts.

In oral testimony doctors should tell the truth, be relevant not arrogant, and not walk out whilst giving evidence. If unclear about any question put, request clarification. Should you require a short break, ask your representative if this can be granted, which is most likely.

Ensure you have a glass of water by your side.

Your lawyer represents you and will be acting in your best interests. As a professional he/she has legal and ethical duties of confidentiality.

The GMC has a code of conduct for council members. In performing their duties, members uphold the seven principles known as the Nolan principles, first identified by the Nolan committee in its 1 May 1995 report on standards in public life. The seven principles are: selflessness, integrity, objectivity, accountability, openness, honesty and leadership. Their corporate responsibilities are as regulators for doctors in the UK, with responsibility for protecting, promoting and maintaining the health and safety of the public by ensuring proper standards in the practice of medicine, as set out in the Medical Act, 1983 as amended.

Council members have a duty to ensure their functions are effectively discharged in the interests of public protection.

The 'standard of proof' is the civil standard which is on the balance of probabilities, as opposed to the criminal standard (a higher one), which is proof 'beyond reasonable doubt'.

22.4 Dishonesty-Forging Patient Notes

The expectation is that a doctor could be struck off, but an apology may lead to a lesser sanction such as suspension or limited suspension.

22.5 Misconduct; Falling Short of Standards

The leading authority on professional conduct is Roylance v The General Medical Council (Medical Act, 1983) before the Privy Council on 24 March 1999; citation 1999 UK PC 16, (2000) 1 AC 311. 1999 3 WLR 541.

The Privy Council upheld the original GMC decision which found the appellant, Mr. Roylance guilty of serious professional misconduct and directed his name be erased from the register. This followed a 74 days hearing before the GMC involving not only the appellant, but two other surgeons, Messrs. Wisheart and Dhasmana. All three charges were inter-related and concerned a number of cardiac operations between 1990 and 1995 on very young children in Bristol Royal Infirmary.

Their Lordships would not interfere with a disposal unless they were satisfied the decision was clearly unjust and were not so persuaded in this instance.

For doctors who may have dyslexia, the employer has to make 'reasonable' adjustments.

22.6   Sexual Relations with Patients

There is an imbalance in the relationship which can be open to abuse, particularly if the patient is vulnerable, in any way, which can lead to some form of sanction.

22.7   Sanctions

The desired effect is punitive, from the least restrictive starting with no further action (which is rare), caution that is possibly 3 or 5 years, reprimand, conditions of practice, 12 months supervised practice then back before the committee, suspension, limited suspension or lastly, struck off.

The Fitness to Practise Rules 2004 (as amended) underpin GMC decisions. Each case will be determined on the facts to ascertain if a doctor's fitness to practise is impaired.

Guidance is not intended to be exhaustive and should be read in conjunction with other relevant guidance such as that produced by the GMC and MPTS, for example 'Good medical practice', 'Sanctions Guidance' and 'Action following referral to the MPTS'.

22.8   Race and the GMC

For the purposes of the Law, the GMC is a 'qualification body' under sections 53 and 54 of the Equality Act, 2010. This is because it is responsible for the registration of doctors. Therefore, when applying sanctions, it is or should be entirely impartial, that is not biased, nor as a body discriminate, nor victimise.

However, concerns have been raised about the disproportionate number of Black, Asian and minority ethnic (BAME) doctors coming before the GMC compared with their white counterparts. Moreover, if there is a white comparator, recent cases have suggested the white Doctor is treated more leniently, as arguably in the 2021 case of Mr. Omer Karim.

The 1994 revelation by Esmail and Everington was that ethnic minority Doctors are 6 times more likely to be investigated than white Doctors. In their article they argue parallels can be drawn between 'structural racism and institutional racism in the NHS we have witnessed to that witnessed in the GMC'.

Currently, 4 in 10 Doctors in the UK are from ethnic minority backgrounds. Without them, the NHS could not function. Yet not only do minority ethnic doctors find themselves referred to the GMC more often, but they can then arguably face further discrimination from GMC processes themselves. In Mr. Karim's case the tribunal said that for aspects of its investigation, it seemed the GMC was *'looking for material to support allegations against Mr. Karim, rather than fairly assessing materials presented'*.

This is despite reports even commissioned by the GMC itself, such as the June 2019, 'Fair to refer' Baroness Helena Kennedy one, specifically about 'Reducing disproportionality in fitness to practise concerns reported to the GMC'. This was independent research conducted by Dr. Doyin Atewologun and Roger Kline with Margaret Ochieng. Its object was to understand why some groups of doctors are referred to the GMC for fitness to practise concerns, more, or less than others by their employers or contractors and what can be done about it.

The reasons for such disproportionality are complex with a combination of micro factors. Methodology was qualitative with 262 participants: issues of culture, age, training, support and leadership underpinning findings and recommendations.

Summarising its introduction, BAME doctors have more than double the rate of being referred for disciplinary proceedings than white doctors. Non-UK Doctors have a 2.5 times higher rate of being referred by an employer compared to a UK graduate doctor, the former who are more likely to be referred to the GMC by their employers or health care providers for subsequent disciplinary action. But independent studies have found no evidence of bias in GMC decision-making; yet concerns remain in the patterns of referrals, notably about doctors who are neither GPs, specialists, nor in training. Overseas doctors are more likely to be referred than UK graduates. Significantly, referrals by employers and healthcare providers into the Fitness to practise (FtP) process are more likely than complaints by the public to be investigated by the GMC.

'Fair to refer' highlighted inadequate induction and support from employers but hopes that doctors will not be unnecessarily probed in the first place, putting the spotlight on the employer, as opposed to regulators or inspectors.

In Pandya B, Singhal P. Insights from GMC's 'Fair to Refer' report, they argue that the real problem may be at Board level, where non-executive members often fail to take their corporate responsibilities seriously and hold the executive to account. They believe that in the absence of an effective mechanism for 'meaningful engagement with clinicians and front-line professionals, the blame culture and the unsupportive mindset may remain unchanged'.

The high-profile case of Hadiza Bawa-Garba unravelled aspects of poor induction, lack of supervision, unsafe staffing and systemic failures; a textbook example of what went wrong. The nurses and junior Doctor were scapegoated by the system. Regarded as a turning point, its subsequent review and recommendations Pandya B and Singhal P laud as a catalyst which changed the fabric of organisational responsibility and accountability.

The four Recommendations from 'Fair to refer' include:

1. Providing comprehensive support for doctors new to the UK or to the NHS or whose role is likely to isolate them (including SAS doctors and locums).
2. Ensuring engaged and positive leadership more consistently across the NHS.
3. Creating working environments that focus on learning and accountability rather than blame.
4. Developing a programme of work to deliver, measure and evaluate the delivery of these recommendations.

22.9   Mr. Omer Karim's Case

On 6 June 2021 the Reading Employment Tribunal (ET) found that Mr. Karim, a urological surgeon, had been treated less favourably during a GMC investigation than a white colleague on the grounds of race. The GMC said it will appeal.

In its landmark ruling the ET held—

We have come to the conclusion that there is a difference in the treatment of the claimant in contrast to Mr. L, a white Doctor. We do not consider that there has been a credible explanation for the difference in treatment—we consider there is evidence from which we could conclude that the difference in treatment of the claimant in comparison with Mr. L and the delay (in dealing with his case) were on the grounds of his race.

We know for a fact that Doctors from minority ethnic backgrounds are already disadvantaged by being referred by their employers to the GMC twice as often as their white counterparts.

Charlie Massey, the GMC's Chief Executive acknowledged that the Organisation had 'lessons to learn' and said they would like to bring transparency to their own processes. Nevertheless, he defended the GMC's decision to appeal against the decision.

The GMC is appealing the outcome of Mr. Karim's case because it believes that the 'tribunal wrongly concludes that disproportionate referrals to the GMC by employers constitutes evidence of direct discrimination in Mr. Karim's case and also that the case of the doctor to whom Mr. Karim was compared differed in key respects. We shall see if there is any error of law in the tribunal's ruling when it goes to the Employment Appeal Tribunal (EAT).

22.10   Implications of the Case

On a personal level Mr. Karim's world 'fell apart', ruining his life and reputation, compelling him to sell his home to fund his battle with the GMC, and live in a Travelodge for 5 years, away from his family after securing part-time employment in Portsmouth.

This compounds the tragedy of Consultant Anaesthetist Sridharan Suresh who committed suicide within hours of receiving notification that he would be facing an interim orders tribunal in 2018. The BMA is supporting legal action by his widow Viji, against the GMC and Dr. Suresh's former employer.

A letter before action to the GMC says that the regulator should have known that there was a real and immediate risk of suicide, and that there were system failures after the GMC failed to take any steps to liaise with Dr. Suresh's employer or the Police to assess his vulnerabilities, despite Dr. Suresh telling his trust how the investigations were affecting him and his family.

Dr. Chaand Nagpaul, BMA Council Chair said (bma.org—25 June 2021) *'the Karim ruling is not only a landmark one having discriminated against a doctor in pursuing an investigation, but that the GMC must ensure fairness for all as it has dented doctors' confidence in its credibility'.*

This case has been seen in the context of a wider picture of discrimination and disadvantage experienced by BAME doctors. Differential attainment in postgraduate exams, poorer or slower career progression, increased levels of bullying and harassment and an ethnicity pay gap; see Discrimination Advice for Doctors 7 September, 2020.

22.11   DEI/Diversity, Equity and Inclusion and the GMC

'Diversity is being invited to the party; inclusion is being asked to dance', Verna Myers told the Cleveland Bar in Ohio, USA. She continued that overcoming prejudice starts with identifying our unconscious biases and trying to rewire our brains to welcome differences and think more inclusively.

'It is harder to crack a prejudice than an atom', in Einstein's words.

The centre for Creative Leadership uses the REAL framework to shift mindsets, behaviours, and practices towards more equitable and inclusive leadership for organisations such as the GMC. The 4-step process framework incorporates:

1. Reveal relevant opportunities
2. Elevate equity
3. Activate diversity
4. Lead inclusively

The GMC has its own Equity, Diversity and Inclusion guide dated 18 May 2021 with targets [3]. This addresses disproportionality in respect of patterns of fitness to practice complaints received from employers in relation to a doctor's ethnicity and place of qualification which they want to eliminate by 2026. They acknowledge black and ethnic minority doctors are twice as likely to be referred. It sets out how the GMC supports DEI in medicine and includes practical support. This is its strategic vision for the foreseeable future.

It stresses their commitment to tackling persistent inequality, central to their corporate strategy for 2021–2025. By 2031 they aim to deal with discrimination, disadvantage and unfairness in under-graduate and post-graduate medical training and education.

There is a BME/Black minority doctors' forum. Any questions can be emailed to them at equality@gmc.uk.org. Members of the forum include the BMA, Indian

Medical Association, British International Doctors, MANSAG/Medical Association of Nigerians across Great Britain and Association of Pakistani Physicians and Surgeons, amongst others. The BME Doctors' Forum raises issues on behalf of BME and international Doctors' networks and acts as a sounding board.

References

1. General Medical Council. Our investigation process. https://www.gmc-uk.org/concerns/information-for-doctors-under-investigation/how-we-investigate-concerns/our-investigation-process
2. General Medical Council. Fair to refer. https://www.gmc-uk.org/about/what-we-do-and-why/data-and-research/research-and-insight-archive/fair-to-refer
3. General Medical Council. Equality, diversity and inclusion. https://www.gmc-uk.org/about/how-we-work/equality-diversity-and-inclusion

Burn Out in Medicine

23

Danielle Williams

23.1 Definition of Burn Out

"Burn-Out" is a familiar phrase used in medicine and with 1 in 3 medics experiencing burn out at any given time [1], it is crucial to understand what it is and how to address it. Burn-out is a syndrome classified in ICD-11 [2] as mental health illness. In ICD-11 [2] it outlines the syndrome as being made up of three components; Emotional exhaustion, an individual's perceived feeling of worthlessness and reduced quality in a professional's work and showed only be applied in reference to occupation. Burn-out being a common occurrence in the medical field, it is important as doctors to identity triggers of burnout, and how to create environment that is conducive to reduce the prevalence of burn out in the health care work force.

Unfortunately, there are not a lot of studies focusing on Urology trainees and burnout in the UK. A joint British and Irish study was conducted in senior Urologists regarding the rate of burnout and associated factors. This study had a total of 575 participants, and the study scored the individual using the three components of burn out. The results showed a mean emotion exhaustion score of moderate and a mean depersonalisation score of moderate. Also, it is significant to note that positions with managerial and leadership roles reported high levels or burn out, the main causes of burnout were the amount of work, administration workload and lack of resources [3].

Doctors spend their careers and lives identifying ill-health and creating appropriate patient-centred management plans for the public but can often fall short when identifying ill-mental health in oneself and colleagues. Recognising burnout amongst medics and one-self is crucial as it can have a direct impact in patient care.

D. Williams (✉)
The Princess Alexandra Hospital, Harlow, UK
e-mail: danielle.williams40@nhs.net

© The Author(s), under exclusive license to Springer Nature Switzerland AG 2022
F. Motiwala et al. (eds.), *When Things Go Wrong In Urology*,
https://doi.org/10.1007/978-3-031-13658-0_23

I would like to highlight that one of the components of burn out being reduced professional efficacy and a having a negative perception of one's role and place in the workforce. This statement details the potential negative impact it could have on patient care. To care for others, we must care for ourselves, and to care for ourselves we must do our part to reduce the likelihood of burn out.

Burn out is classified as a syndrome conceptualised by emotional and physical fatigue, disinterest, and negative view of one's occupation and reduced professional efficiency secondary to chronic work stress (WHO 2019). Burn out is driven by external and internal stressors which lead to physical exhaustion and emotional depletion. External stressors being the environment around you e.g., a busy ITU ward, a demanding bed manager or patient complaints. Internal stressors are usually created by the expectation of oneself e.g., staying late instead of handing over jobs, or feeling guilty because of patient outcome which you could not have changed [4].

Mental ill health is not unique to medicine, with employers in UK spending a total of nearly £26 billion each year to support staff with mental ill health. It was found in a report written by the National Institute of Clinical Excellence (NICE), that promoting the mental well-being can be of economic benefit to employers with better staff retention, less absences, better work efficacy and increased staff satisfaction. For the National Health Service (NHS) to experience these benefits, they too should prioritise employee mental health [5].

A recent qualitative study analysing the work-life balance in junior doctors, identified a low morale within doctors in training who had felt exploited and dehumanised by their employer. The high-demanding career of a junior doctors can often lead to individuals neglecting their own personal welfare. This can be attributed to trainees delivering a high performance at work whilst simultaneously competing for training post with portfolio boosters, Royal College Examinations and attending conferences. This can leave a little space in their lives for personal fulfilment, which in turn can lead to maladaptive coping mechanism, creating a strain on both patient and colleague relationships thus risking patient care in the long-term.

Doctor burn out is evident in the UK, with rising number of Foundation Year 2 doctors not applying to higher speciality training, around 79% in 2019, and choosing to have gap years or leave medicine all together, and with those taking a sabbatical from medicine has increased from 4.6 to 13.6%.

23.2　Contributing Factors to Burn Out

To reduce the likelihood of having burnout, it is important to understand the triggers that are present in the career of medicine that can precipitate burn out. Contributing factors in the medical field to name a few; the poor work-life balance, the pressure to see more patients within strict time frames and inefficiencies in administrative task. The triggers of burnout in medicine which are generally similar for all specialities can be placed in three categories: the culture of medicine, practice inefficiency and personal resilience. The culture of medicine can at times promote an unhealthy lifestyle an improper work-life balance and encourage resilience instead of promoting self-care and personal self-growth. To promote wellness within medicine, it is important to foster good relationship with colleagues, compassion not only for patients but for our colleagues as well. Hence, Mess committee and social events outside work with colleagues should be encouraged. To promote efficiency of practise good and modern infrastructure is crucial and can have a direct impact not only on patient care but on the workload of doctors. Personal resilience is made up from one's environment to improve physical, emotional, and professional well-being. Developing personal resilience is down to supports systems one has around them at home, work and financially [4].

23.3 Recognition of Burnout

It is important to recognise Burn-Out in oneself and colleagues, it presents self in the following ways:

- Poor Performance
- Reduced Creativity
- Exhaustion Physically and Emotionally
- Headaches/Stomach Aches
- Cynicisms at work

23.4 Mindfulness

Throughout this chapter we have learnt about what burn out is, why it is so prevalent in medicine and the triggers of burn out. We have previously also touched on the fact there are triggers outside your control therefore we must optimise how we preserve one's mental health whilst working in such a difficult career.

A pre-post observational study with 93 participants who are doctors partook in an 8-week Mindfulness course of 2.5 h a week and a 7-day retreat. The course was provided 11 times over 6 years and it showed improvement in healthcare providers' emotional exhaustion, depersonalisation, personal accomplishment, and overall general mental health well-being [6].

Professor Mark Williams, former director of the Oxford Mindfulness Centre, says that "mindfulness means knowing directly what is going on inside and outside ourselves, moment by moment." The idea of mindfulness is to be present in what you're doing, so you do not fixate on the issues and stressors in your life but give yourself a break to enjoy yourself and be in the moment.

To be more mindful takes practise, and you will have to slowly build it to a habit. Take time each day to spend 2 min being mindful. Become more aware of your thoughts and try to label emotions. For example, one thought could be "I am stressed about an upcoming exam". Acknowledge that emotion is anxiety and sit with the emotion. Studies show that labelling your emotions reduces the psychological distress and enables you to understand your emotions better, making it easier to deal with the emotion.

Mindfulness can be hard to practise at first for some individuals. When they practise to be mindful, one can focus on the task at hand whether it is washing-up, yoga or running but once they have stopped the activity, they can have thoughts that rush into their mind and overcrowd their mind. When this does happen it's important to realise that that these thoughts have not been addressed before. It can be described as "thought traffic" in a busy carpark. The thought traffic being the thoughts that race through your mind, the carpark your mind, and mindfulness is the gate allowing cars out. The more you practise mindfulness, the more the carpark gate is open to allow thought traffic out of the carpark. It can take you mind some time unclog the thought traffic occurring in your mind however the more you practise mindfulness the more affective can be [4].

It is also important to understand mindfulness can happen in a multitude of ways through meditation, exercise, and music etc. Currently there are a lot of apps that you can use to encourage yourself to be mindful. Also, gratitude journals and apps are similarly taking the time to appreciate the positivity in one's life.

There is also the GAIN method. It is an acronym for Gratitude, Acceptance, Intention and Non-judgment. It does not take a lot of time, usually only 3 min. It can be done whenever and is probably easiest to do when you wake up. Start by taking deep breaths in and out. First state what you are grateful for, for example "I am grateful for my physical health, the privilege of being a doctor and contributing to patient care etc." Acceptance is to acknowledge we all have pain and suffering in our lives, that it is important to acknowledge this and accept that you did not cause it, and that you cannot change it but accept it exists. Intention is to acknowledge that you have power to think and react to the situation around you, acknowledge what you can control and what you can do. It is about being empowered to make change in your own life that will benefit you. Non-judgement is about accepting that not everything has to be labelled as good or bad and can just exist. The world in its magnificence and greatness does not need to be compartmentalised and being indifferent to things can be more useful and soothing [4].

By applying this technique, you can be more prepared when an external stressor hits such as an encounter with a rude colleague. Instead of labelling them as rude, take some deep breaths, remember what you are grateful for, accept what you cannot change, and know it is not your fault or responsibility to fix them. Remember your intent for the day and don't judge the person for being rude as the person does not need a label, which in turn can reduce the emotion inside of you.

The precipitants to burnout are rife in the medical profession. The external and internal factors that drive burn out are hard to avoid. Hence it is important to understand what the factors are, so we can work together to reduce it. On national a level there does need to be some change to systems, infrastructure, and training posts so that it encompasses and promotes good mental health for all doctors. On a personal level it is important to protect yourself and keep yourself healthy by using a technique to reduce that chance of burn out in oneself, and to ensure that you maintain a good work life balance. It is important to implement a good work life balance otherwise it could be detrimental to one's health.

References

1. De Hert S. Burnout in healthcare workers: prevalence, impact and preventative strategies. Local Reg Anesth. 2020;13:171–83.
2. ICD 11. https://icd.who.int/.
3. Chen H, Liu F, Pang L, Liu F, Fang T, Wen Y, Chen S, Xie Z, Zhang X, Zhao Y, Gu X. Are you tired of working amid the pandemic? the role of professional identity and job satisfaction against job burnout. Int J Environ Res Public Health. 2020;17(24):9188.
4. Hammer GB. Mindfulness and GAIN: The solution to burnout in medicine? Paediatr Anaesth. 2021(1):74–9.
5. Imo UO. Burnout and psychiatric morbidity among doctors in the UK: a systematic literature review of prevalence and associated factors. BJPsych Bull. 2017;41(4):197–204. https://doi.org/10.1192/pb.bp.116.054247. Erratum in: BJPsych Bull. 2017;41(5):300.
6. Goodman MJ, Schorling JB. A mindfulness course decreases burnout and improves well-being among healthcare providers. Int J Psychiatry Med. 2012;43(2):119–28.

NHS Whistleblowing

24

Hanif Motiwala, Faiz Motiwala,
and Sanchia S. Goonewardene

Any doctor or staff working in NHS has duty to raise concern about care if a patient is harmed or being harmed. This also applies to adult social care. This may involve patent safety issues or when a patient's dignity is compromised. This is called whistleblowing. There are various examples of it. For example, patients left in their own urine and excreta without dignity, patient's food and water intake not cared properly or patients even being shouted or being physically attacked. This also involves poor care standards of not giving medications when due, or practices involved where patients are discriminated against e.g. for being disabled, due to their race and so forth.

In the UK, whistleblowing is defined as the raising of concerns in the public interest by a worker, whether to their employer or externally through a range of designated channels (the chief of which are termed 'prescribed persons') [1]. Ultimately, workers may make a wider disclosure, for example to the media but there is limitation to it with good reason.

24.1 Is it Safe to Raise Concern and Be Whistle Blower?

The history of NHS whistle blowers is littered with injustice and suffering as many have suffered, bullied, harassed, sacked and driven to despair.

H. Motiwala
Department of Urology, Southend University Hospital, Southend-on-Sea, UK

F. Motiwala
Queen Elizabeth Hospital, London, UK
e-mail: Faiz.Motiwala@nhs.net

S. S. Goonewardene (✉)
Department of Urology, The Princess Alexandra Hospital, Harlow, UK

F. Motiwala et al. (eds.), *When Things Go Wrong In Urology*,
https://doi.org/10.1007/978-3-031-13658-0_24

1. Dr. Steve Bolsin raised concerns about mortality in the Bristol paediatric heart surgery scandal, which resulted in a Public Inquiry report in 2001. He reported being ostracised and famously decided to leave the country [2]. He left the UK to live and practice in Australia. This was a famous case and an initial one to emerge, as a lot of paediatric mortality and morbidities were ignored, and whistleblowers were being bullied and harassed.

2. Raj Mattu, the former cardiologist at Walsgrave Hospital in Coventry, exposed a crisis of overcrowding and patient safety at his unit in 2001. Mattu's reward was a suspension and a decade-long struggle before he was eventually exonerated. This was despite the CQC publishing a report later in 2001 describing it as the 'worst ever' patient safety report they had produced for any Trust, confirming an 'excess death rate' of 60% [3, 4].

3. The rogue breast surgeon Ian Paterson subjected more than 1000 patients to unnecessary and damaging operations over 14 years before he was stopped, an independent inquiry found. Paterson was free to perform harmful surgery on mainly female patients in NHS and private hospitals because of a culture of "avoidance and denial" in a "dysfunctional" healthcare system where there was "wilful blindness" to his behaviour. The inquiry found that victims were "lied to, deceived and exploited" by Paterson, who is serving a 20-year jail sentence imposed in 2017 for wounding with intent and unlawfully wounding nine women and one man whom he treated between 1997 and 2011. Several whistleblowers raised the concern over the years who were ignored and even bullied [5].

4. Dr. Linda Reynolds, a GP, raised the alarm over Harold Shipman. The Public Inquiry by Dame Janet Smith commented on issues of disbelief, which whistleblowers often encounter [6].

5. BBC News published the following story in 2021, where an inquiry was commenced in 2019 by the Police, into 456 patient deaths after receiving opiates between 1987 and 2001 in Gosport War Memorial. No charges have been made for them. The Police began the inquiry after the Gosport Independent Review Panel found there was a "disregard for human life" at the hospital in Hampshire. Most whistle blowers were ignored. An independent investigation, led by Kent and Essex Serious Crime Directorate, is still currently reviewing millions of pages of evidence. About 150 detectives and staff are expected to be involved in the probe [7].

6. In a public inquiry by Sir Francis Roberts in the Mid Staffordshire disaster, it was revealed how the Trust Managers and those with Governance responsibility ignored all warnings and concerns raised by the staff and how the staff were bullied and cover ups were fully exposed.

Sir Francis reported in the Mid Staff public inquiry that 'there are many reasons why people may feel reluctant to speak up in any industry. For example, they may be concerned they will be seen as disloyal, a 'snitch' or a troublemaker'. According to Sir Francis:

two particular factors stood out from the evidence gathered: fear of the repercussions that speaking up would have for an individual and for their career; and the futility of raising a concern because nothing would be done about it.' The legislation which theoretically provides protection for whistleblowers is contained in the Employment Rights Act 1996, as amended by the Public Interest Disclosure Act 1998, commonly known as PIDA. Where a worker makes a protected disclosure, he/she has a right not to be subjected to any detriment by his employer for making that disclosure.

For a number of reasons this legislation is limited in its effectiveness. At best the legislation provides a series of remedies after detriment, including loss of employment, has been suffered. Even these are hard to achieve, and too often by the time a remedy is obtained it is too late to be meaningful.

In Robert Francis Mid Staffordshire Public Inquiry report, he included a recommendation that obstruction of whistleblowing should be a criminal offence. However, he distanced himself from such a position in his later *Freedom to Speak Up* review. This review has been criticised for not providing strong enough recommendations. Vitally, the review let control remain with the employers. This is certainly a precarious approach when such serious matters involving life and death allows the defendant to also be the judge, jury and executioner.

24.2 Current UK Law to Protect Public Interest

Current UK whistleblowing law is flawed. Even one of individuals who helped to draft the current law, Lord Touhig, recognised this. The law does not compel investigations into concerns and confers poor legal protection. Reprisals against whistleblowers have devastating effects. Amends and promises to whistleblowers have not been fulfilled which sets a poor precedent and sends a poor message of support towards whistleblowers and current NHS staff.

24.3 Doctors in Training and their Whistleblowing Protection

Junior doctors are at forefront therefore can see deficiency in service. There may be gap in rota for proper patient safety and care. A recent case gained significant press attention, of that involving Dr. Chris Day in [Day v Lewisham NHS Trust and Health Education England]. Dr. Day raised several concerns to both the trust and Health Education England (HEE) regarding staffing on the medical wards while working an ICU shift. He later submitted an Employment Tribunal claim was submitted for unfair dismissal and whistleblowing detriment i.e. unfair treatment due to raising whistleblowing concerns. During the initial hearing, HEE successfully argued that it did not have a duty to protect whistleblowing junior doctors suffering any detriment as it was not their employer—yet it then raised the question—who had the duty to protect the whistleblower? This decision was appealed by Dr. Day and subsequently overturned. This general case was fought and dragged on for 4 years causing significant stress, with significant costs before being eventually withdrawn after 6 days in a tribunal commencing October 2018. A statement withdrawing his claims, agreed by all three parties, was read out. This raised significant awareness and prompted the need for several changes to improve whistleblowing protection including that from the BMA [8], however this is certainly a space worth watching.

24.4 GMC and Whistleblowing

The GMC guidance states the following:

> All doctors have a duty to raise concerns where they believe that patient safety or care is being compromised by the practice of colleagues or the systems, policies and procedures in the organisations in which they work. They must also encourage and support a culture in which staff can raise concerns openly and safely [9].
>
> Doctors in training may also raise concerns with the GMC about their place of training. However only those with a working relationship with the organisation about which they are raising concerns will be protected from detriment or dismissal under whistleblowing legislation. The GMC has established on-line reporting of such complaints and concerns. One can use confidential helpline as well. The number is **0161 923 6399** [10].

While the GMC do say they will help and support whistleblowers, they have also sadly failed to protect whistle-blowers in the past, and in many cases in fact supported the Trust who went after the whistleblowers. The GMC have pursued against whistleblowers on the behest of the Trust where concerns were raised. This has been fully exposed in Sir Anthony Hooper's inquiry in detail [11].

24.5 Duty of Candour and Harm

Duty of Candour is where every healthcare worker must be honest and truthful to their patients when something goes wrong. It applies as Professional duty of candour as per the GMC where patients or their representatives require an explanation of what went wrong, an apology offered when appropriate, and all efforts directed for remedial support. Above all doctors have ethical and moral duty to be transparent.

The statutory duty and regulation apply to all organisation registered with CQC. NHS organisations have to report safety incidences and 'never events'. The moderate or severe harm and prolonged psychological harm is also included in the act. This rate of this is increasing, and particularly there should be consideration of clinical harm in the recent period of COVID-19 and the post COVID scenario where routine and even cancer care was delayed across the nation. Patients waiting for such length of periods are at an increased risk of harm and reviews of this should occur.

Errors occur every day in clinical practice across the world. It may result in mild to even severe harm, but as a doctor it is part of our duty and responsibility to be honest and transparent.

24.6   My Summary and Conclusion

Currently fear still runs high amongst NHS staff to raise concerns. It is much more difficult for a trainee. No one wants to be called troublemaker. According to CQC, the majority of hospitals across the country have safety issues. Despite this, whistle-blowers are not listened to or protected. In an ideal world they should be heralded as Champions of Public Interest.

Having been a whistleblower myself, I have suffered simply for raising concerns. False allegations were raised and eventually I was reported to the GMC along with my colleague who won the case in Employment Tribunal against the GMC for discrimination, the first such case pursued in Tribunal against GMC.

There is an ethical and moral dilemma for every doctor, and the failure to protect whistleblowers has resulted in a type of complex culture system where it simply remains a paper exercise. People may have differing views however until the spirit of openness and transparency is firmly rooted in our health system, the status quo will not change.

References

1. NHS England. Raising a concern with NHS England. https://www.england.nhs.uk/ourwork/whistleblowing/raising-a-concern/. Accessed October 2021.
2. BBC News. Bolsin: the Bristol whistleblower. http://news.bbc.co.uk/1/hi/health/532006.stm. Accessed October 2021.
3. Chowdhury S. Press release from Dr. Raj Mattu's legal team. https://sharmilachowdhury.com/2016/02/10/press-release-from-dr-raj-mattus-legal-team/. Accessed October 2021.
4. The Guardian. Dismissed NHS whistleblower who exposed safety concerns handed £1.22m. https://www.theguardian.com/uk-news/2016/feb/04/dismissed-nhs-whistleblower-who-exposed-safety-concerns-handed-122m. Accessed October 2021.
5. Ian Paterson and failure by oversight bodies. https://minhalexander.com/2017/06/01/ian-paterson-and-failure-by-oversight-bodies/. Accessed October 2021.
6. The Shipman Inquiry. 2nd report. Chairman Dame Janet Smith DBE. https://assets.publishing.service.gov.uk/government/uploads/system/uploads/attachment_data/file/273226/5853.pdf. Accessed October 2021.
7. BBC News. Gosport hospital deaths: inquiry reviews 15000 death certificates. https://www.bbc.co.uk/news/uk-england-hampshire-56404256. Accessed October 2021.
8. Rimmer A. BMA will support legal fight of whistleblowing junior doctor Chris Day. BMJ. 2021;374:n1731.
9. General Medical Council. Raising and acting on concerns about patient safety. https://www.gmc-uk.org/ethical-guidance/ethical-guidance-for-doctors/raising-and-acting-on-concerns/part-1-raising-a-concern#paragraph-7. Accessed October 2021.
10. General Medical Council. GMC policy on whistleblowing. 2018.
11. General Medical Council. The handling by the General Medical Council of cases involving whistleblowers. Report by the Right Honourable Sir Anthony Hooper to the General Medical Council presented on the 19 March 2015. https://www.gmc-uk.org/-/media/documents/Hooper_review_final_60267393.pdf. Accessed October 2021.

Index

© Springer Nature Switzerland AG 2022
F. Motiwala et al. (eds.), *When Things Go Wrong In Urology*,
https://doi.org/10.1007/978-3-031-13658-0

Printed in the United States
by Baker & Taylor Publisher Services